Narrativ

Karen In

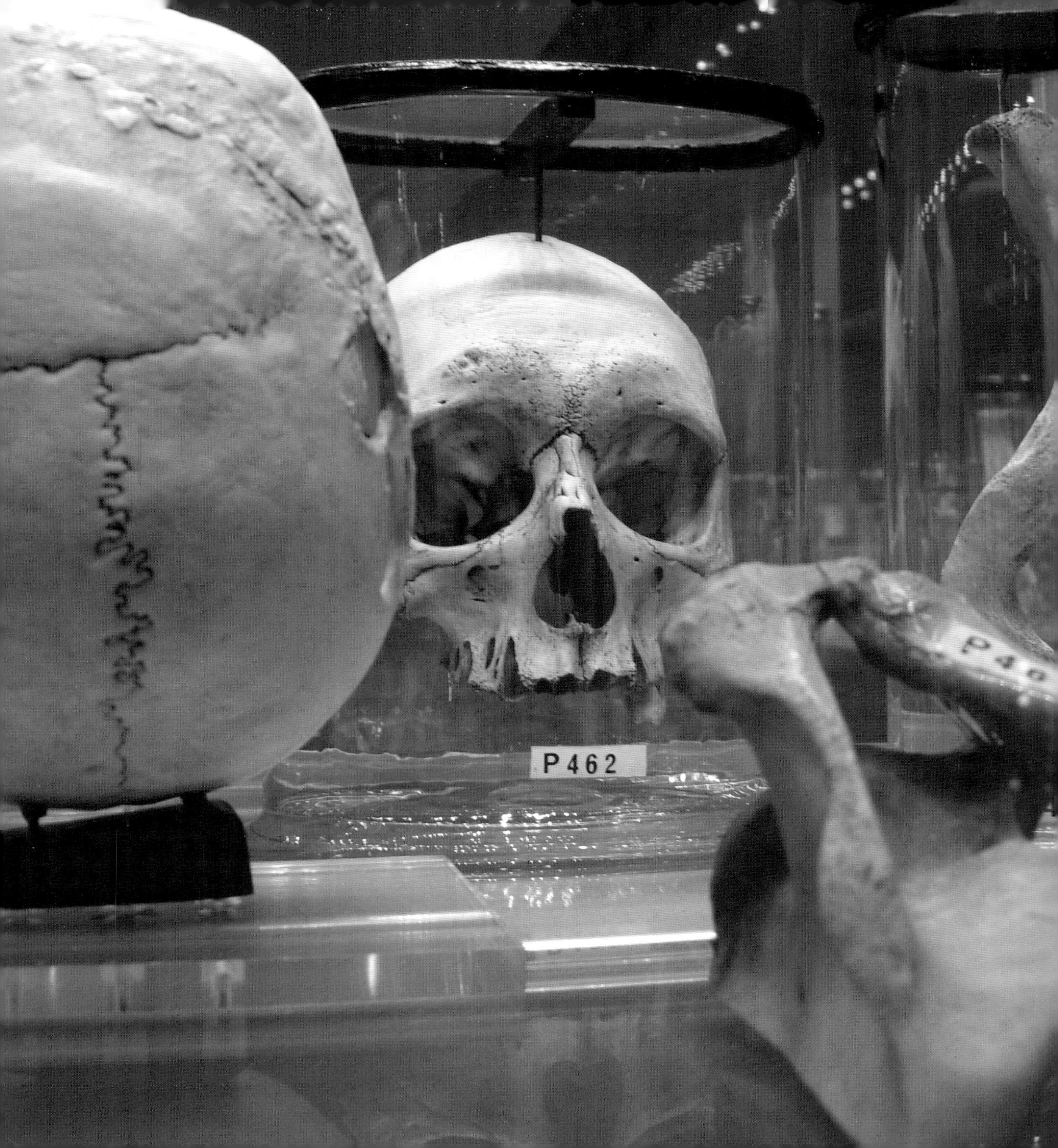
P462

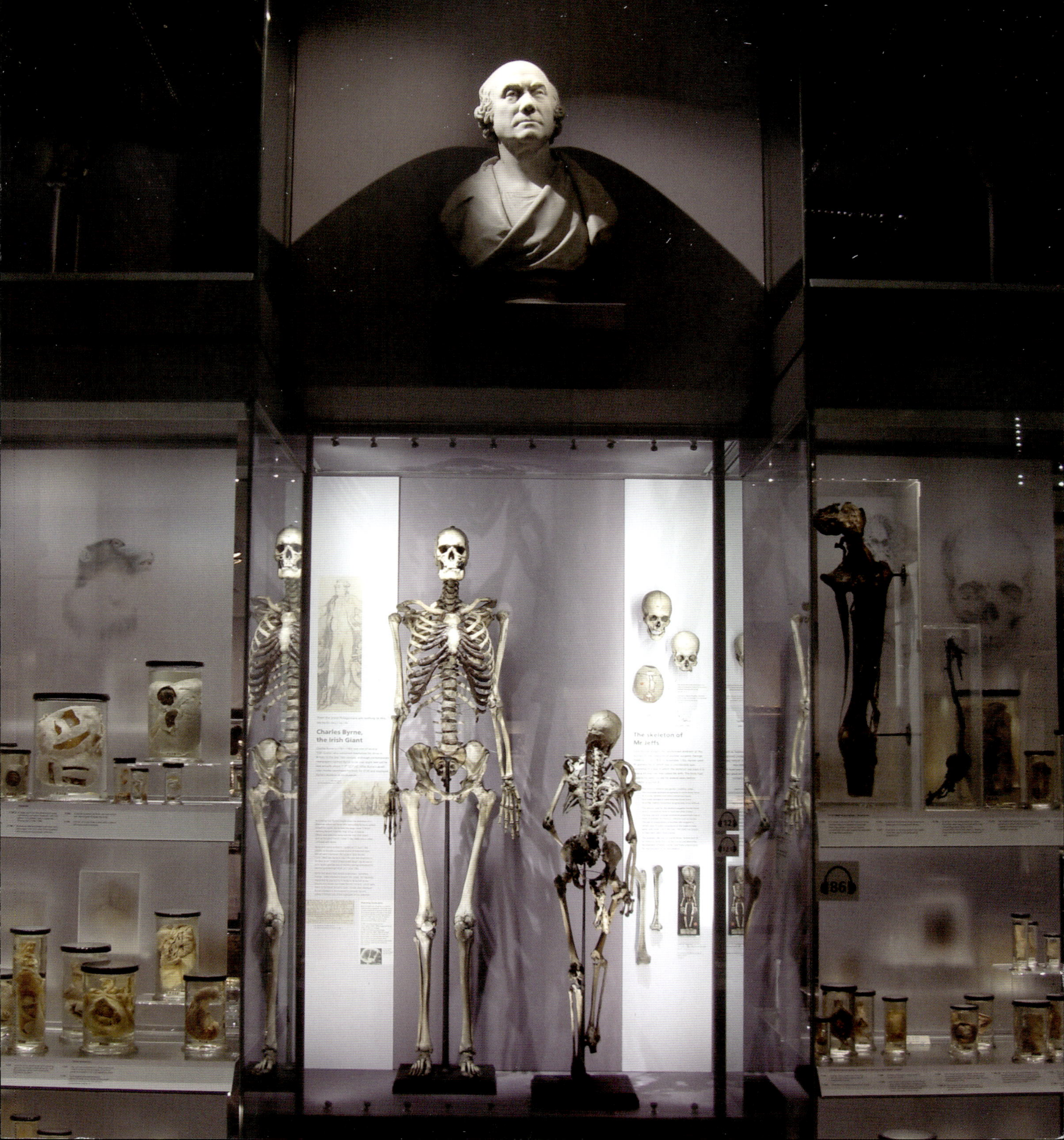
Charles Byrne, the Irish Giant
The skeleton of Mr Jeffs
86

Emotion and Identity in John Hunter's Museum

Simon Chaplin

Emotion and Identity in John Hunter's Museum

Simon Chaplin

To untrained eyes a pathological specimen is a barren, lifeless thing. Detached and disembodied, it is an object made by hands skilled in the craft of unpicking the fabric of the human body. It is presented for the appreciation of discerning medical eyes, trained to delineate diseases which penetrate organs or traverse planes of tissue. The specimen speaks, too, with a medical voice; in terms that are anatomical, pathological or histological, the lingua franca of the clinician or biomedical scientist. Most of all it is anonymous. Its accompanying case history may lay bare the most intimate details – reveal age and gender, health and habits, dissect a life with the same dispassion that has been brought to bear on the body – but the narrative is always impersonal, the patient is not named, and their voice has no place.

Have emotion and identity ever been part of the museum of pathology? For Michel Foucault, it is precisely the removal of these uncontrollable qualities that characterises modern clinical medicine. In the hospitals of post-revolutionary Paris, he locates an epistemic shift that changed the way doctors saw their patients, through the emergence of a penetrating 'clinical gaze' which turned individual patients into medical objects. Not surprisingly, the pathological specimen – by definition dissected and abstracted, stripped of context – has become an emblem of this cultural change. Others have looked back further in time, and across the Channel, to see evidence for the birth of the clinical gaze in the charitable hospitals and private anatomy schools of Georgian London. The emergence of the anatomist as exemplary figure and the demise of the patient as individual have been seen as inextricably linked. In John Hunter – the archetype of the surgeon-scientist – some have seen the origin of an exclusive medical authority that still, today, denies the patient a say – a 'fearful symmetry' between Hunter and his successors, as Ruth Richardson so eloquently describes it.

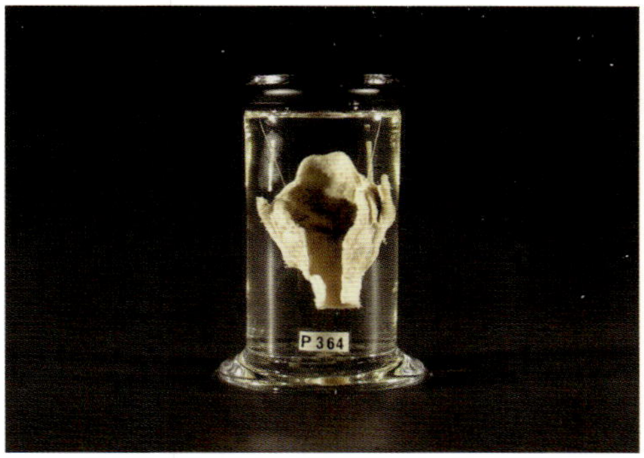

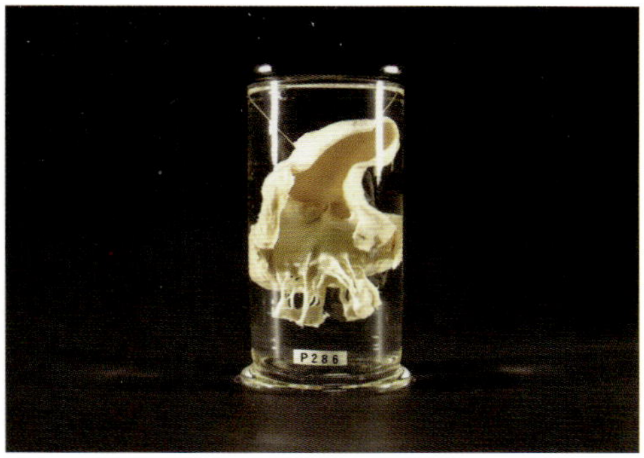

Revealing the patient's voice in John Hunter's collection, invoking identity to engender emotion, can therefore be seen as a political act. It is a way of highlighting the origins of the clinical gaze in order to deflect or refocus it, and to bring the modern patient back into the picture. But the fact that these identities are there to be recovered should make us pause. Why do we know their names – Richard Bulstrode, Mrs Adams, Marianne Harland and more? Was Thomas Thurlow – a Bishop! – subjected to the same indignity as the author Laurence Sterne: disinterred, 'resurrected', and spirited away, only to be revealed in the cold light of day on the dissector's table? We know that John Hunter was, like his many contemporaries, dependent on an illicit trade in cadavers conducted by London's 'resurrectionists' or grave-robbers. His case-books contain plenty of dispassionate accounts of dissections performed upon anonymous bodies, some secured through hospitals, others from work-houses or the gallows at Tyburn. 'In 1759 I stripped the bones of an old woman that died in St George's Hospital', begins one such record, 'I knew nothing of her history'. Yet his notes also include many details of patients with whom Hunter was more familiar: people of rank, of wealth, and of power, whose stories are preserved, and whose own voices can be heard in the records of their final illnesses. Hunter's knife cut through the social and economic divides of Georgian society, bringing together clerics and criminals, politicians and paupers, merchants and tradesmen. In an essay on post-mortems in Britain in the 17th-century, David Harley has argued, *pace* Foucault, that such histories are evidence of a more multivalent political economy, in which patients, rather than practitioners, often held sway. If, as Norman Jewson has suggested, the 18th-century witnessed the disappearance of the 'sick man' from medical practice, then Hunter's case-books suggest that this was a gradual process, and one that was the result of a careful process of negotiation, rather

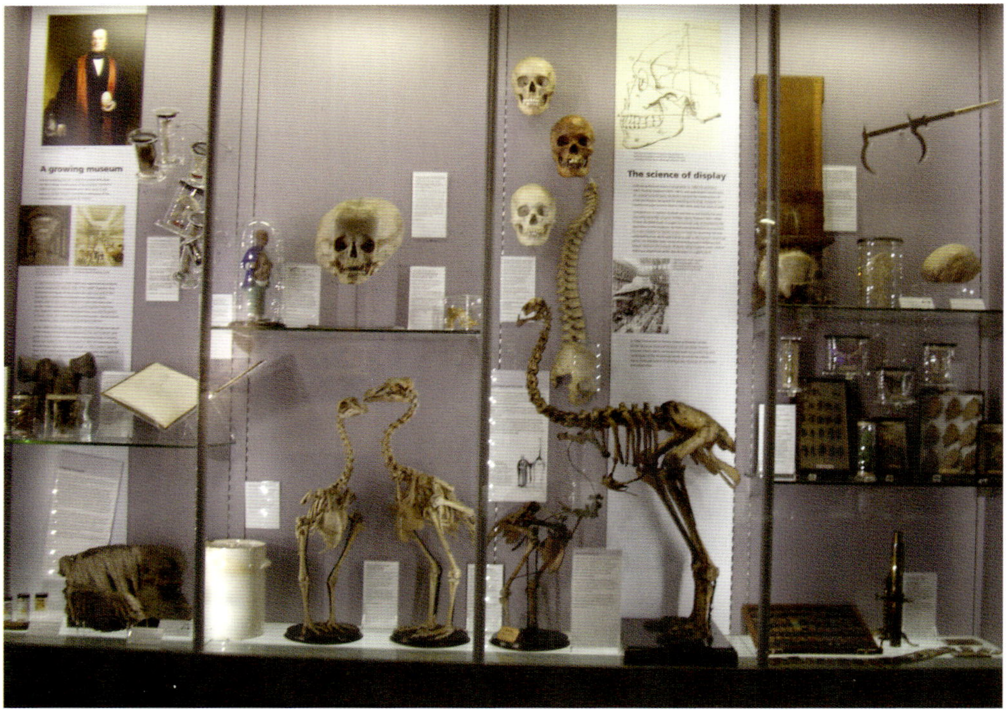

simply than the imposition of a new model of medical authority.

Written case histories formed part of this process. Published in learned journals, and often re-circulated in literary magazines or reported in the press, they were accessible to and read by a much wider audience than we might imagine. For the historian Thomas Laqueur, they form part of a broader literary genre, the 'humanitarian narrative', which used the plight of the patient to create a 'moral imperative' for actions that appeared beyond the pale – harsh physic, radical surgery, and post-mortem dissection among them.

A calculated appeal to the sensibilities and sympathy of readers, these narratives invited readers to put themselves in the place of the sufferer, to appreciate their travails and their stoicism in the face of adversity. Employing the patient's voice lent these narratives a rhetorical urgency. By emphasising the role of the patient or their family as the instigators of dissection, they also portrayed it as a duty that served both private interest and the public good.

It was not only in print, however, that patients spoke from beyond the grave to sanction the act of dissection. As the

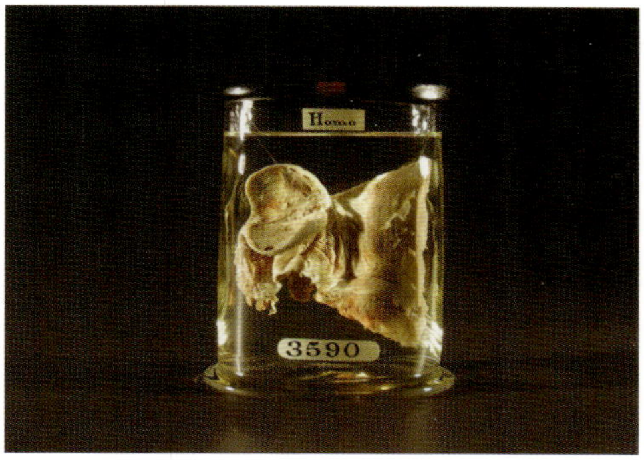

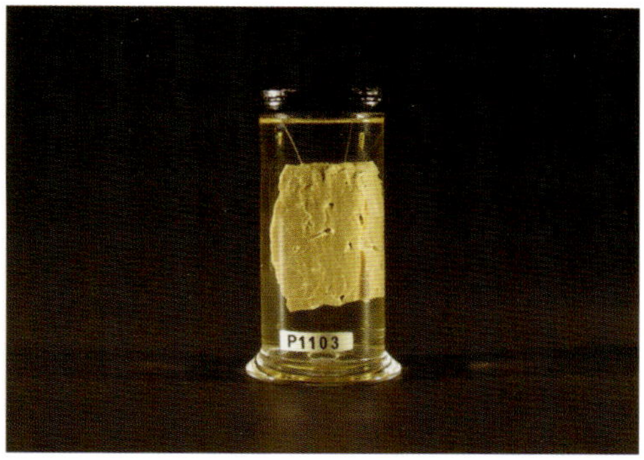

cases of Harland, Bulstrode, Johnson, Thurlow, Adam and Hunt show, Hunter preserved parts of many of the bodies he dissected, 'putting them up' as 'wet preparations' pickled in spirits of wine, or desiccated and varnished as 'dry preparations'. Like his many rivals, Hunter measured his success through his museum, a repository that came to house over thirteen thousand preparations by his death in 1793. Normal and morbid, human and animal, the body parts in Hunter's collection testified to the range of his interests, the scope of his practice and – the ever-present connection – the skill with which he wielded his knife. From 1785 his collection was housed in a purpose-built structure behind his house in Leicester Square, a three-storey edifice with lecture theatre, meeting room and gallery combined. Here, his preparations jostled for attention, pots of limpid spirit in which were suspended pieces of sculpted tissue, rendered vivid by injections of coloured wax. It was, according to a syllabus for Hunter's lectures, 'a most instructive school for the student', a material encyclopaedia of disease which demonstrated Hunter's mastery over his craft. It was also, however, a place in which Hunter could make his work presentable to a wider audience. Each Saturday in May, Hunter opened his museum to the public – three Saturdays for gentlemen, one Saturday for ladies – and it is likely that it was viewed at other times, especially by the 'literati' who gathered in Hunter's house each week for the salon hosted by his poet wife, Anne.

Among those who viewed the museum and its serried ranks of morbid bodies was the antiquary and author Horace Walpole. Plagued by gout, he joked blackly to a friend that the 'chalkstones' from his suppurating knuckles might find a home in 'Mr Hunter's collection of human miseries'. His choice of words suggests a different way of looking at Hunter's preparations, not with the restrained and emotionless medical gaze, but with a lively literary eye that invested objects with their own narratives – something that

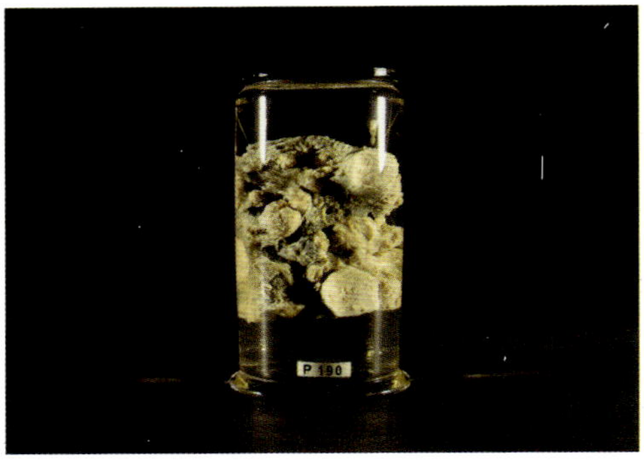

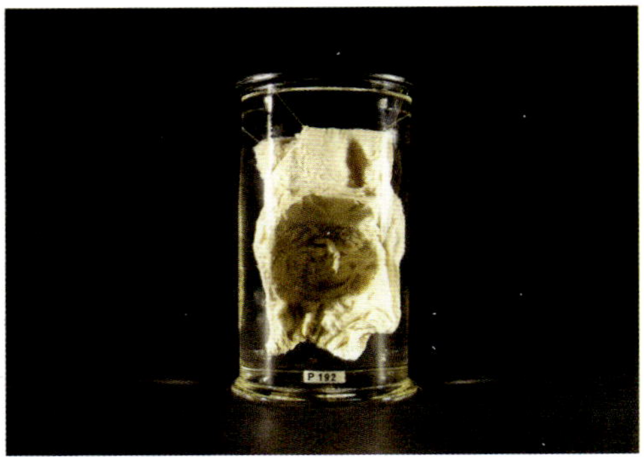

characterised Walpole's own work as a writer and collector. For a well-read spectator, Hunter's museum offered a rich source of novel sensation, a physical embodiment of the sublime terrors of contemporary gothic fantasies such as William Beckford's *Vathek* (1786), with its abundance of 'hump-backs [and] wenny necks'. The imagined ability of inanimate preparations to speak their own stories echoed the literary vogue for 'novels of circulation' – the titillating narratives of everyday objects that provided a scurrilous glimpse into the private lives of others, such as Charles Johnstone's *Adventures of a Guinea* (1760). Such spectators did not, however, need to rely on imagination alone to conjure personal tales from the body parts on show in Hunter's museum. Many preparations were physically inscribed with the names of patients, painted on to the tops of jars or carved in to lead tags suspended around their necks. Case-histories too were kept with the pots, allowing spectators to read for themselves the accounts of the patient's last days. No doubt these too offered some voyeuristic appeal: it is hard not to imagine the pathos evoked by Mary Hunt's lonely suicide, for example.

Nevertheless, naming preparations encouraged spectators to see them as bits of real people, and by doing so gave agency and authority to the dead. The preparation from Thurlow was labelled 'Cancerous Rectum. Late Bishop of Durham' – a brief caption which conveyed not only the organ and its illness, but also the patient's social position. In the appended case history, Hunter's role in the case was revealed. Having seen a succession of physicians who prescribed violent purges but gave no relief, Thurlow 'sent for' John Hunter, who applied the expertise gained through dissection to the diagnosis of his patron: Immediately, upon introducing my finger up the rectum, near three inches, I felt a rising, forming a ridge...This was so familiar a feel to me, that I at once pronounced it to be what is commonly called a Cancer.

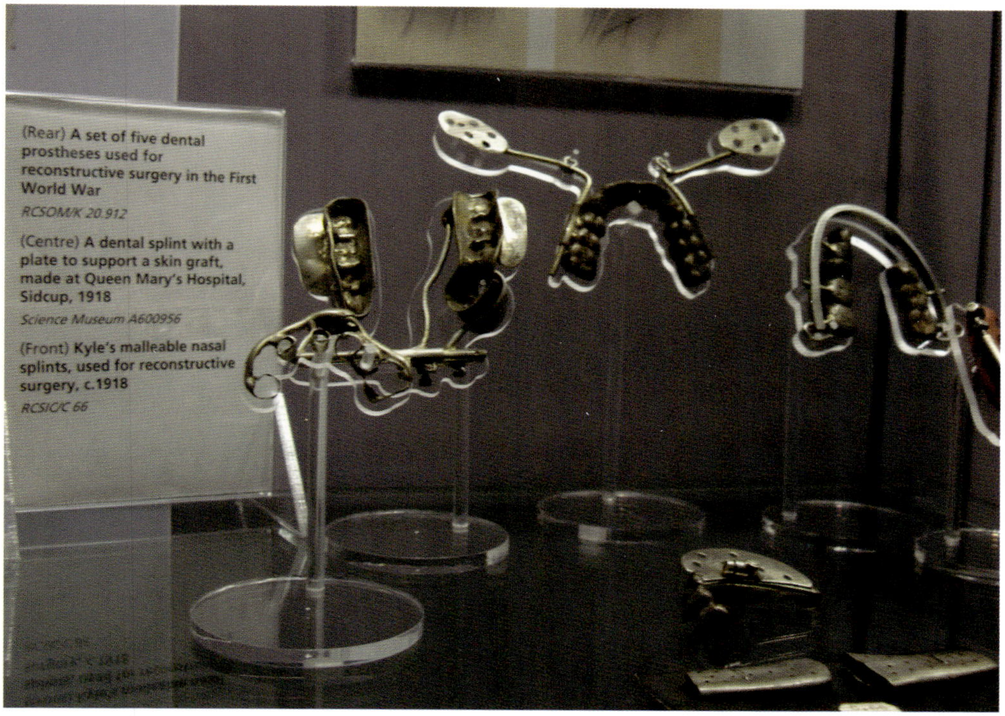

On studying the specimen two centuries later, the eye is still drawn to the mass of the tumour, rendered self-evident through its centrality, as a silent testimony to Hunter's trained touch. Through the case history and inscribed name, the preparation was imbued with a narrative, spoken through the patient's own body. Crucially, Hunter's authority in Thurlow's case-history was constructed not in opposition to the patient, but rather as his servant, and his defender against anatomically ignorant physicians.

It is a measure of Hunter's success in enlisting the bodies of his patients as witnesses to his skill that, after he died, his collection was purchased by the government and presented to the Company (shortly to become the Royal College) of Surgeons. The Hunterian Collection has been treasured by the College ever since, the physical and symbolic presence around which the body-corporate of surgeons has shaped itself. But as the fortunes of surgeons have waxed, so the status of the patient, as represented through Hunter's preparations, has waned. Within the museum, preparations were stripped of their identities: names scrubbed from the tops of jars, and excised from their accompanying case-histories.

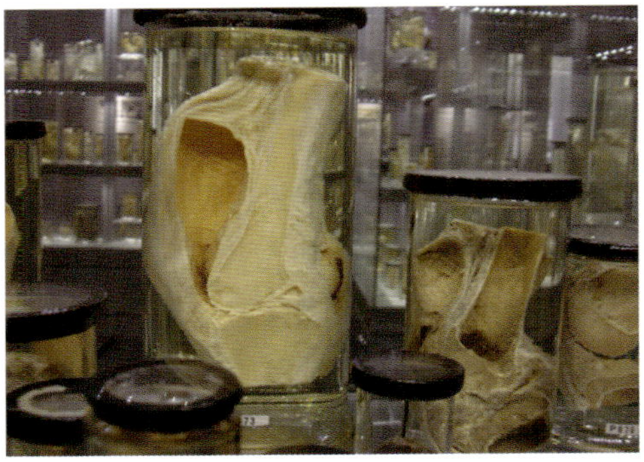

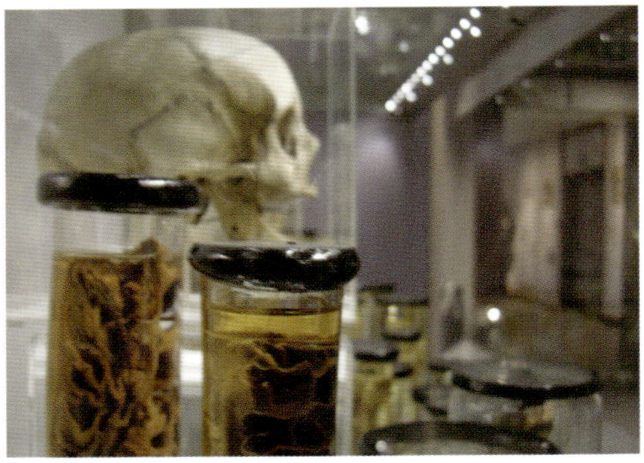

The preparations – singular and identifiable – became specimens, preserved for their medical value as illustrations of types, rather than as exemplary individuals. Karen Ingham's installation, *Narrative Remains*, is not simply the product of artistic invention, but is something much more: an act of revelation, and of reinstatement.
By resurrecting the dead and reinvesting the patient with their story, we recover a sense of the museum as it was: a place of lively stories told through morbid remains.

Allen, Elizabeth, et al., eds. 1993. *The Case Books of John Hunter FRS*. London: Royal Society of Medicine.

Blackwell, Mark. 2004. The it-narrative in eighteenth-century England: animals and objects in circulation. *Literature Compass* 1:1-5.

Cohen, Emily Jane. 1995. Museums of the mind: the Gothic and the art of memory. *ELH* 62 (4):883-905.

Foucault, Michel. 1989 [1973]. *The birth of the clinic: an archaeology of medical perception*. Trans. A. M. Sheridan. London: Tavistock.

Harley, David. 1994. Political post-mortems and morbid anatomy in seventeenth century England. *Social History of Medicine* 7(1):1-28.

Keel, Othmar. 1998. Was anatomical and tissue pathology a product of the Paris clinical school or not? In *Constructing Paris medicine*, ed. C. Hannaway and A. La Berge, 117-183. Amsterdam: Rodopi.

Mack, Ruth. 2008. Horace Walpole and the objects of literary history. *ELH 75* (2):367-387.

Richardson, Ruth. 2001. *Death, dissection and the destitute*. 2nd edition. London: Phoenix, 409-428.

Simon Chaplin is Director of Museums and Special Collections at The Royal College of Surgeons of England. A zoologist and historian of medicine, he has recently completed a doctoral thesis on John Hunter's 'museum oeconomy', and is currently working on an illustrated companion to the Hunterian Collection.

Film Stills

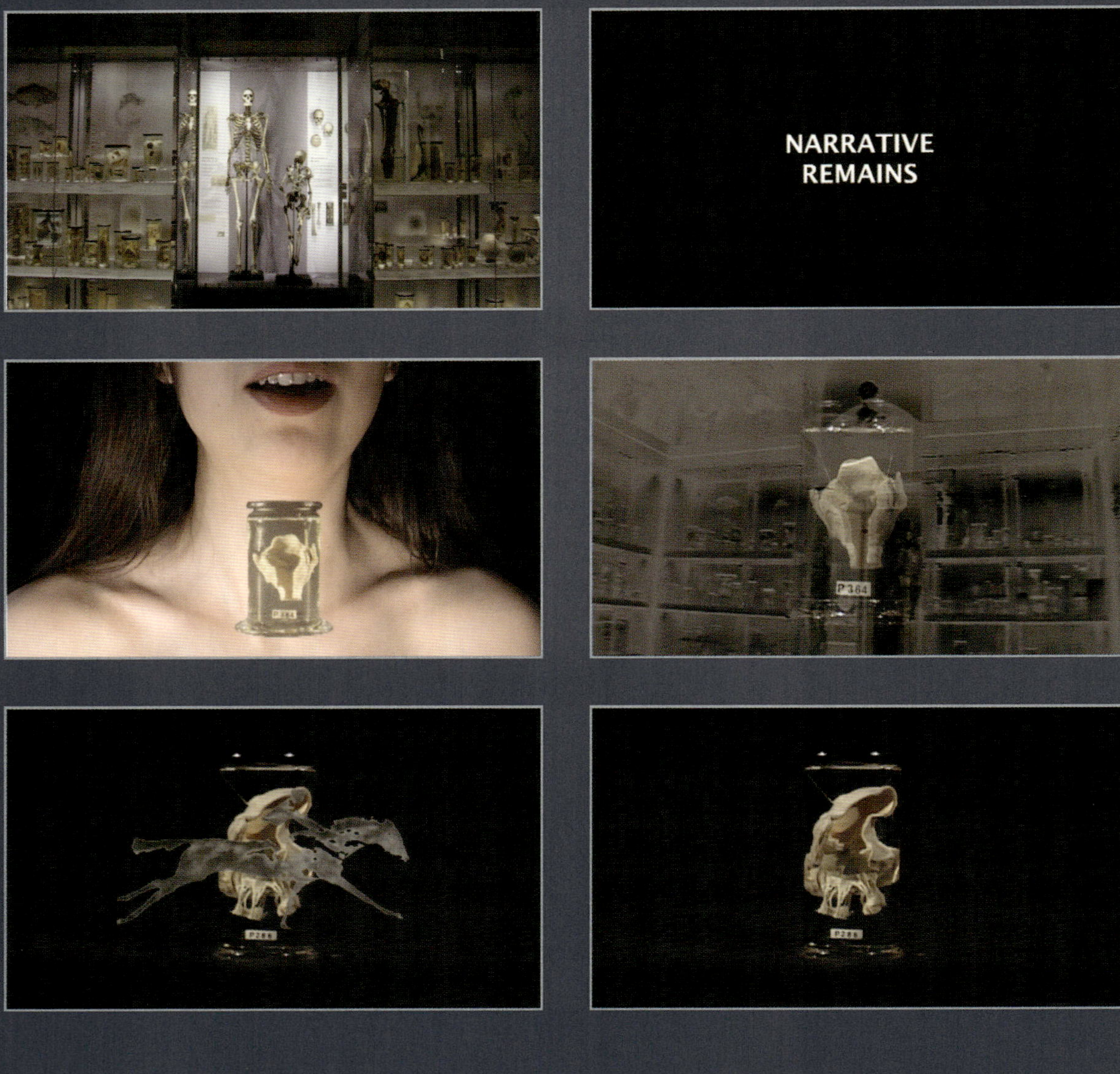

Film stills

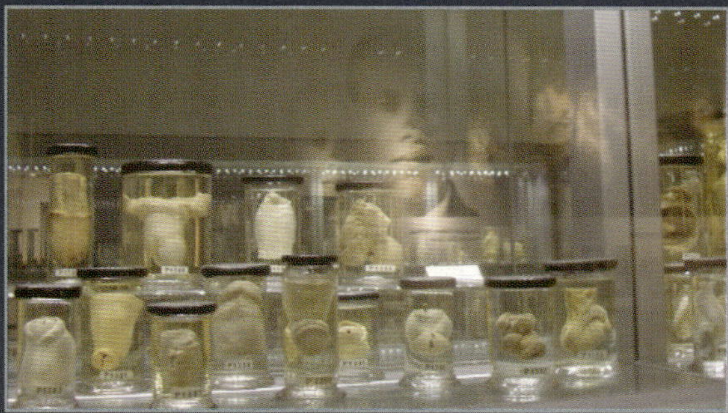

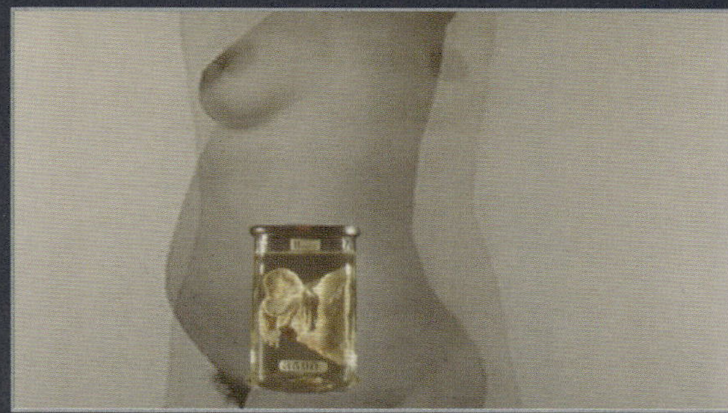

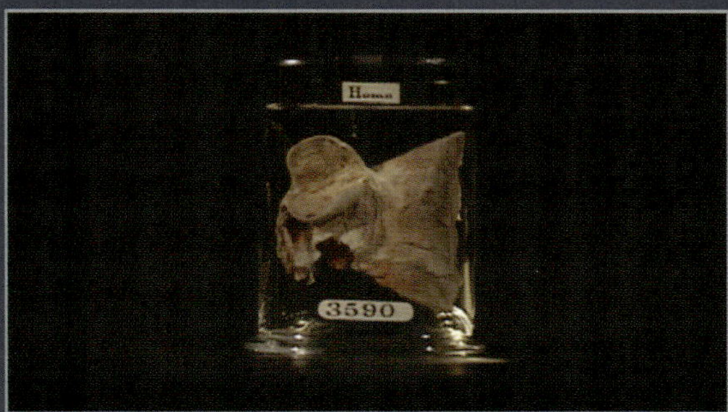

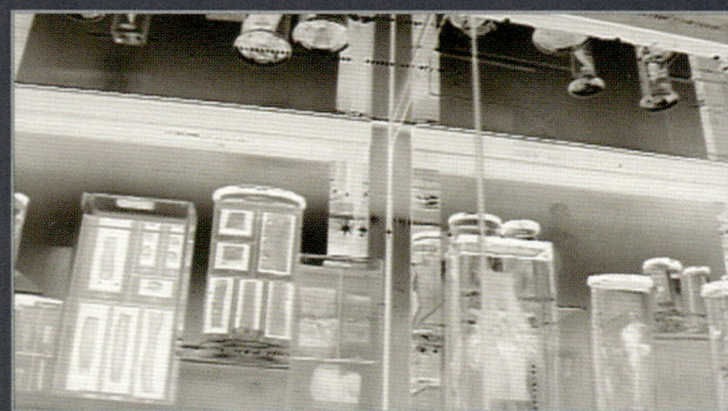

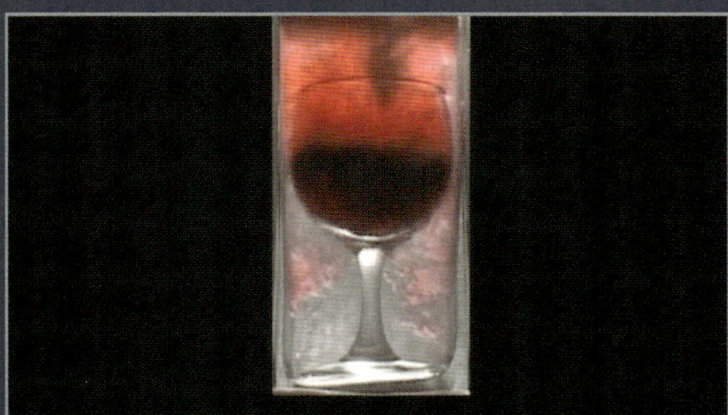

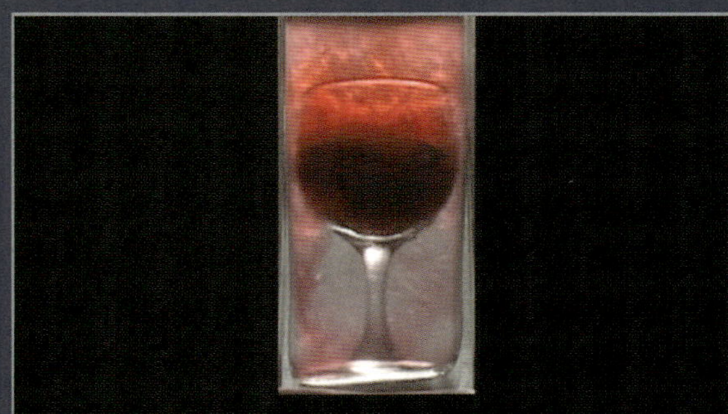

Film stills

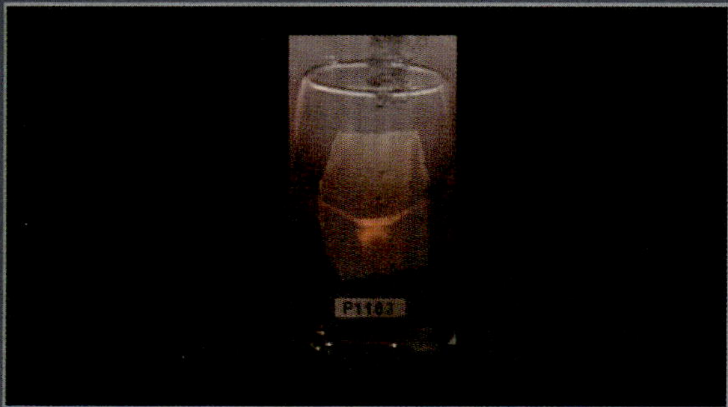
P1183

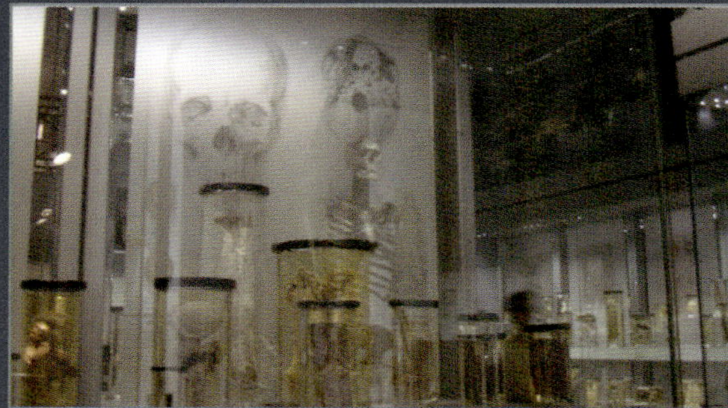

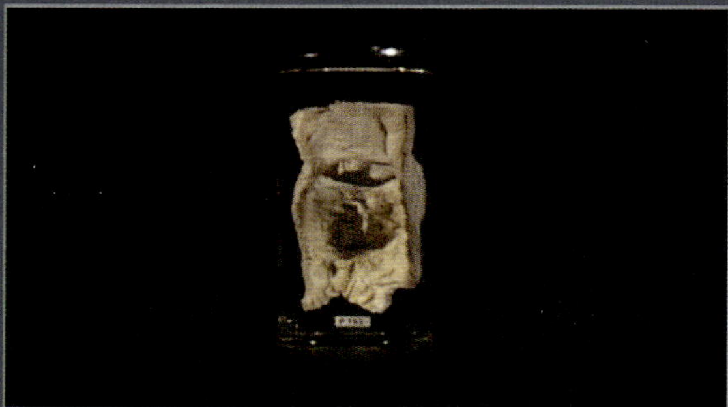

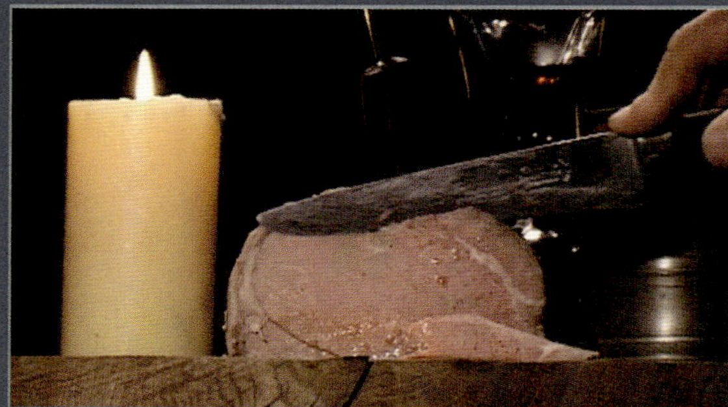

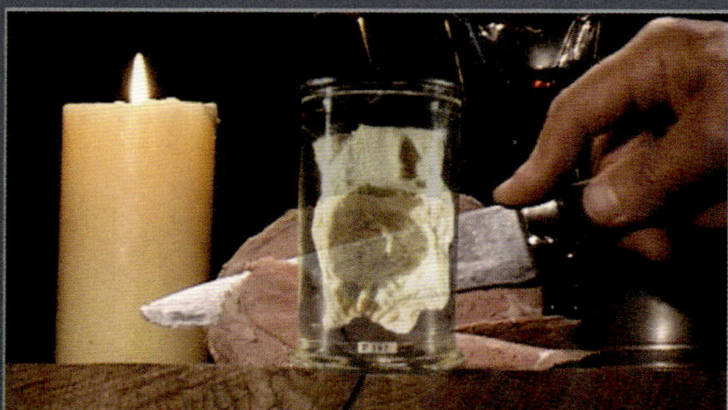

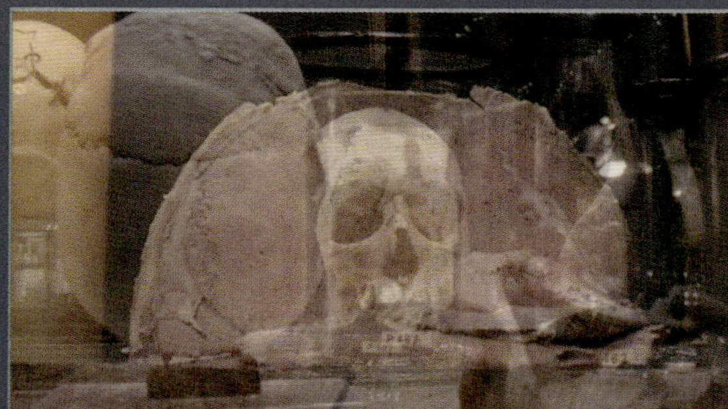

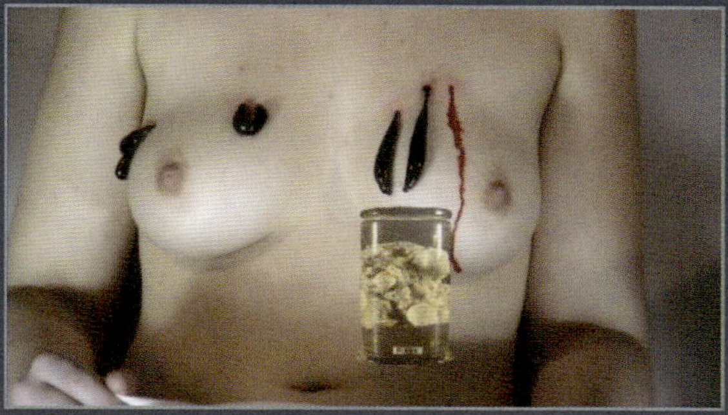

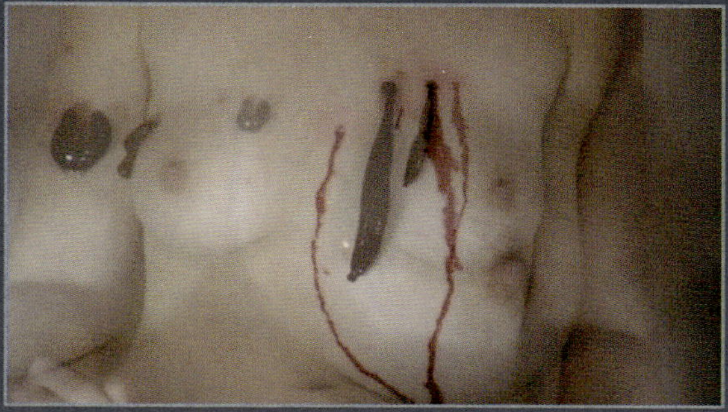

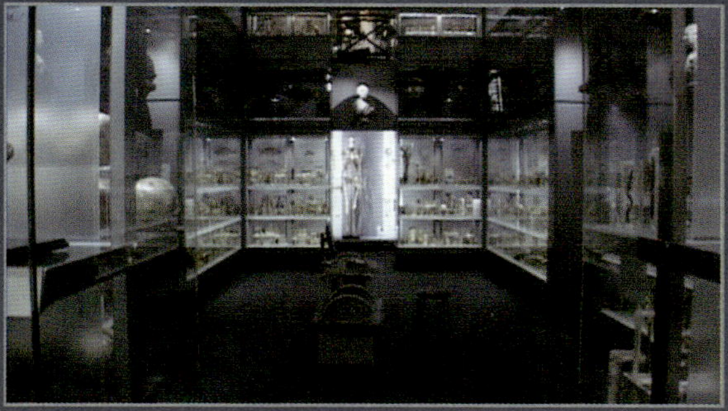

Film stills

All The Dead Voices

Karen Ingham

All The Dead Voices
Karen Ingham

Estragon: All the dead voices.
Vladimir: They make a noise like wings.
Estragon: Like leaves.
Vladimir: Like sand.
Estragon: Like leaves.
(Silence)
Vladimir: They all speak at once.
Estragon: Each one to itself.
(Silence)
Vladimir: Rather they whisper.
Estragon: They rystle.
Vladimir: They murmer.
(Silence)
Vladimir: What do they say?
Estragon: They talk about there lives.

Samuel Beckett, *Waiting for Godot*, 1954

I find myself alone in the space of the crystal gallery, the sudden silence momentarily disconcerting. Gradually, within the stillness, I sense the presence of the dead. If I listen carefully will I hear their whispers? In front of me is the obstetrics collection. Bay 24, Shelf 3. Jar after jar of tiny infants in various stages of development. All the dead voices: what do they say?

Five little girls, their mouths open in unspoken speech, hang suspended in a formula of formaldehyde. Their hands are nearly touching, as if about to play a game together. But these hands will never touch. These are lives that were stilled before they began, and their words will remain unspoken. I scan the display case for the interpretive text boards that might provide further information, an insight perhaps, to these poignant tableaux. I learn that these female quintuple foetuses are the product of human generation from a premature birth at about five months. But the brief contextualising statement tells me nothing more of the human

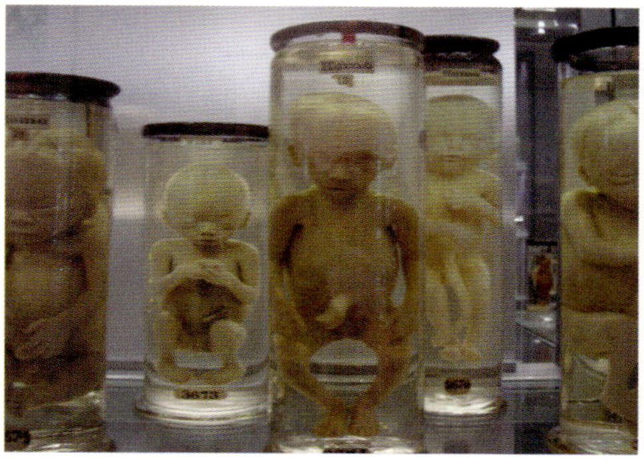

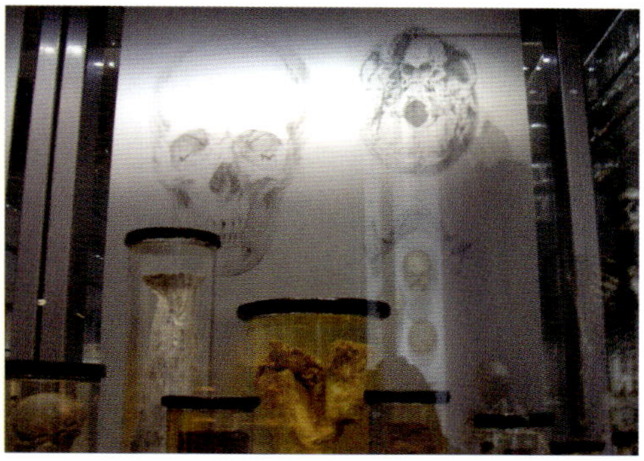

story behind these morbid remains. I consult the Royal College of Surgeons online database for the Hunterian collection. This yields the following information:

“Two of the quintuplets were still-born; the other three died shortly after delivery. They were born to a mother in Blackburn, Lancashire in 1786. A local surgeon called John Hull attended the birth. In his report Hull describes how he was allowed to take the bodies of the foetuses, but was not permitted to take the placenta, which was burnt in accordance with local custom. He sent the preserved bodies to London and they were placed in John Hunter's museum.”

This proves to be more rewarding. These first snippets reveal a more human side to the story, a story where local custom was powerful enough to override the wishes of important men of science. As the case notes progress, I read that the mother's name was Margaret Waddington, born in 1765, and a female patient of John Hull, and that “the mother of the above children, who was 21 years of age, and had previously borne a single child, conceived again in December 1785, and on April 24th, 1786 brought forth these five foetuses, the time of delivery occupying 50 minutes. Each foetus was enclosed in its own amnion, and was attached by a separate umbilical cord to a common undivided placenta…”

So now we have a name, a place and a date, and the outline of a narrative from which we can begin to surmise, to conjecture, to identify with. And here they are now, in front of me, with their melancholy beauty. No doubt they served their post-mortem purpose well, further informing the nascent medical science of eighteenth century obstetrics, insights that would have been put to good use in helping to understand, and thus prepare, for future multiple gestations and deliveries.

I have no difficulty in understanding their ‘purpose’; this is not the first

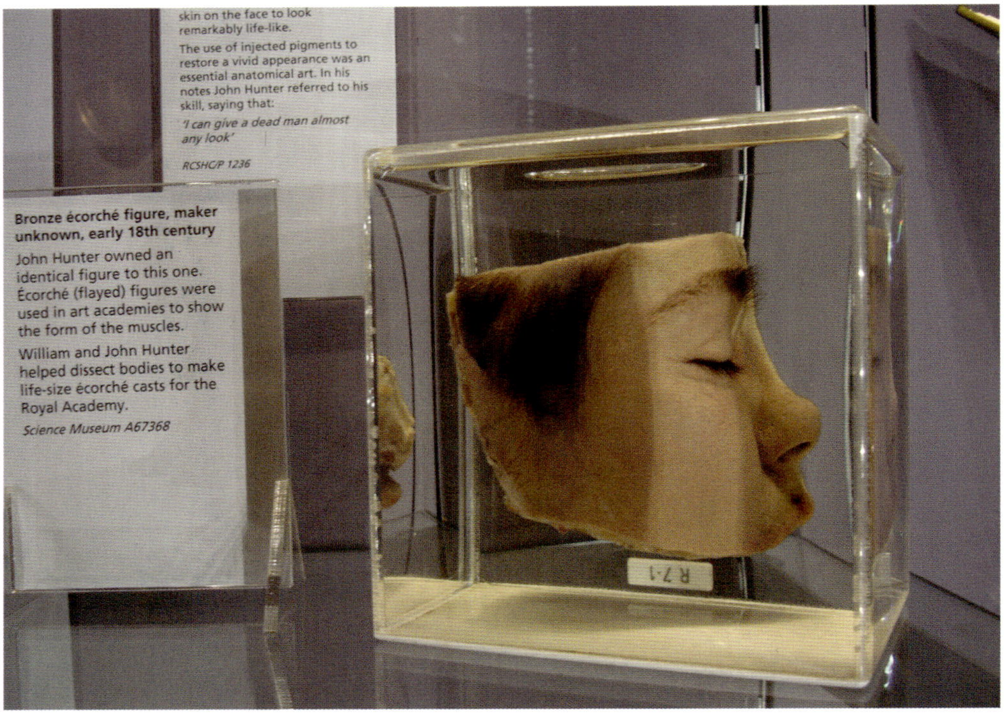
skin on the face to look remarkably life-like.
The use of injected pigments to restore a vivid appearance was an essential anatomical art. In his notes John Hunter referred to his skill, saying that:
'I can give a dead man almost any look'
RCSHC/P 1236
Bronze écorché figure, maker unknown, early 18th century
John Hunter owned an identical figure to this one. Écorché (flayed) figures were used in art academies to show the form of the muscles.
William and John Hunter helped dissect bodies to make life-size écorché casts for the Royal Academy.
Science Museum A67368
R.7.1

collection of anatomical specimens I have studied, and it is unlikely to be the last. I have observed medical students performing dissections on cadavers and understand the need for first hand knowledge of the body. I would want my organs to be used wherever possible in the event of my death, a death that I would hope would be fully investigated and accounted for through the process of the post mortem autopsy. But I also comprehend the profound social and ethical implications of these processes and the public misgivings and misunderstandings of anatomical and pathological investigation and procedure. Museums like the Hunterian are purposefully committed to a programme of public engagement with these complex and topical issues. By working in collaboration with the Hunterian's director Simon Chaplin, it is hoped that projects such as *Narrative Remains* may help to stimulate informed discussion around the retention, preservation, study and display of preserved body parts.

But *Narrative Remains* is not just about public engagement: it is about the power of art to transform and provoke: to bring to life what at first glance appear to be still, dead objects; to animate the inanimate. The project

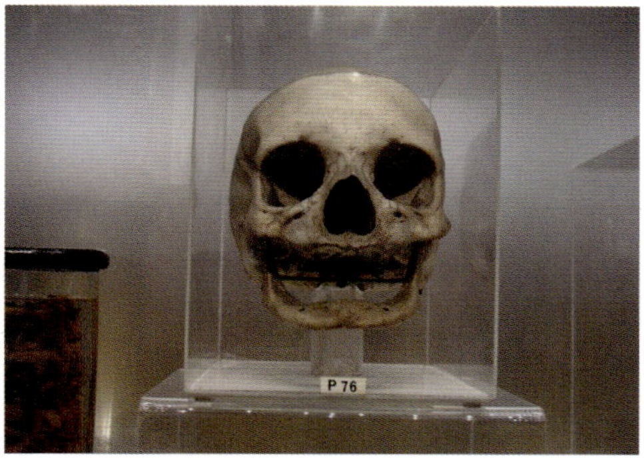

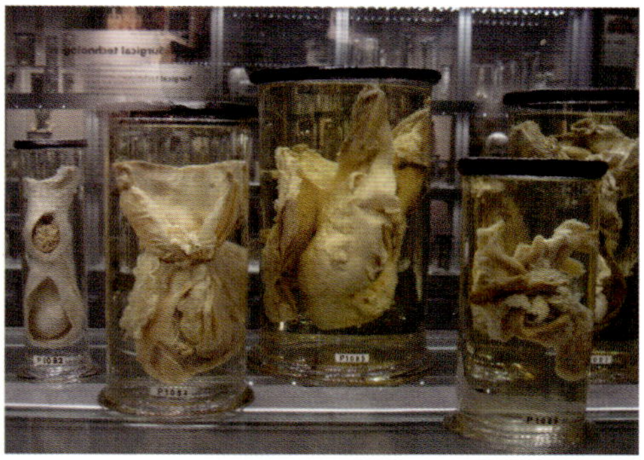

takes its cue from a long tradition of narrations by the speaking dead. The seventeenth-century play *The Anatomist*, by Edward Ravenscroft, proved to be incredibly popular with the audience of the day, notably, as Jonathan Sawday suggests (1995:45) because of "...the macabre presence on the stage of a corpse which comes to life and protests against its own anatomisation." A contemporary performance piece that plays on Ravenscroft's drama is Mike Tyler's *Holoman: Digital Cadaver* in which the digital ghost of a dissected criminal haunts his own theatre of anatomy as a disembodied spectre, questioning his decision to allow his executed body to be dissected and reconstituted as the world's first 'digital cadaver'. This notion of the speaking dead is part of the 'Corpse Poem' tradition, described by Diana Fuss (2003:1) as "…poetry not about the dead but spoken by the dead."

The proliferation of post-mortem television dramas over recent years would suggest that the corpse poem is back in fashion, and the idea of a corpse or even a dismembered head speaking from beyond the grave has become a more widespread narrative device. But what of the actual organs of the dead: how can a heart or lung possibly narrate a story? It is relatively easy to identify with the quintuplet female foetuses, as five little girls as they are identifiably human, premature and undeveloped but nonetheless 'whole'. I can imagine their lives were they to have survived, and I can re-embody their narrative and project it back onto their small, still corpses. There is a poignancy to object number RCSHC/3681 that imbues the hermetically sealed pot with a universal humanity.

But that same sense of humanity may be found in a single organ if perceived as a metonym. For example, object number RCSHC/364 the throat of Marianne Harland, a young woman famed for her musical talents and the beauty of her singing voice. Her death

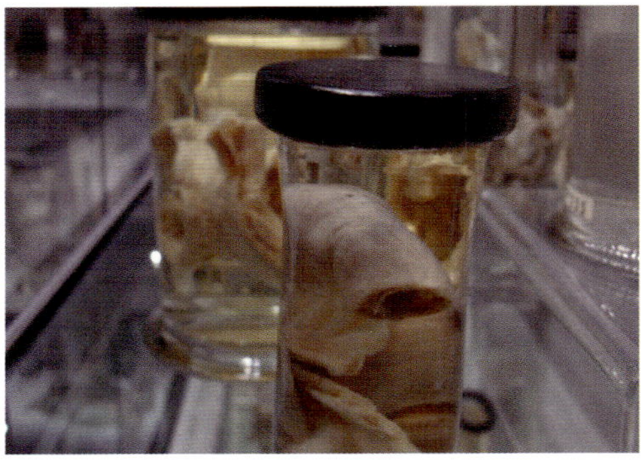

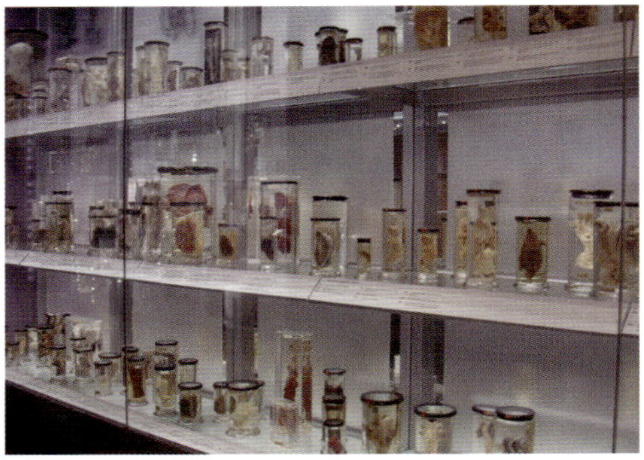

was particularly poignant as she lost first her famed voice, and soon after her life, as a result of tuberculosis. Her oesophagus, larynx and trachea now hang suspended and forlorn and many visitors could easily pass by these seemingly modest displays without ever knowing the human story behind them.

Or the case of Mary Hunt, a young domestic servant who committed suicide through poisoning when she suspected she was pregnant. Her uterus and fallopian tubes are all that is left to tell her story, and as such, they come to represent the whole of her, emblematic, just as Marianne Harland's throat symbolises a voice silenced and a life cut short.

I know these facts, meagre as they are, because there are limited case notes in the RCS database, and it is in part the availability of historical background that determines my selection of the remains I chose to narratively 're-embody'.

But it is more than this. Walking through the collection, the anatomical objects meticulously preserved and displayed, the gleaming glass jars in the spectacular atrium reflecting amorphous forms and shapes, it isn't difficult to sense a ghostly presence, wholly imagined but potent nonetheless, emanating from particular displays.

Perhaps, if I listen hard enough, I may hear a whisper from the throat, or a murmur from the uterus, and I may imagine what these lives were like, what these stories reveal. So this is how I come to find myself in the calm, still space of the Hunterian Crystal Gallery. Sometimes listening, sometimes imagining, always projecting, stories and images, knowledge and wonder.

All the dead voices.
What do they say?

Beckett, Samuel, 1954. *Waiting for Godot*. New York: Random House

Edward Ravenscroft's *The Anatomist* was first first performed in Lincoln's Inn Fields (the present day site of the RCS Hunterian Museum) in 1696

Sawday, Jonathan, 1995. *The Body Emblazoned: dissection and the body in Renaissance Culture*. London and New York: Routledge

Mike Tyler's *Holoman: Digital Cadaver* was first performed at Utrecht Festival a/d Werf in 1997

Fuss, Diana, 'Corpse Poem' in Critical Inquiry, Vol.30, No.1, Autumn 2003. Chicago: University of Chicago Press

Karen Ingham is an artist, writer, curator and a Reader in Art and Science Interactions at the Dynevor Centre for Art, Design and Media at Swansea Metropolitan University. She has an MPhil from the University of Wales for her research into photography and the memento mori and a PhD for her investigations into creative collaborations in the anatomical theatre.

Specimen Narratives

The Uterus | RCSHC/3590

Mary Hunt

"I didn't want to do it but once my employer knew I was pregnant I'd be out on the street and as good as dead anyway. There was nothing for it, not for the likes of a poor girl like me. The poison did its job and I thought that was an end to it but the surgeon John Hunter thought different. He opened me up and poked here and there exclaiming this way and that with fancy names in Latin I couldn't make head nor tail of. But he seemed to find me of interest, which was gratifying, for gentlemen of his class never found me of interest when I was alive. They'd look right through me, which is funny really, as that's what you're doing now, looking through the bits of me, here in this glass jar. Looking where the baby was, too small to really see or even feel, but he knew just what had come to pass. And now here I am, in a place with other bits of mothers and babies, so it's almost like I'm part of a family after all."

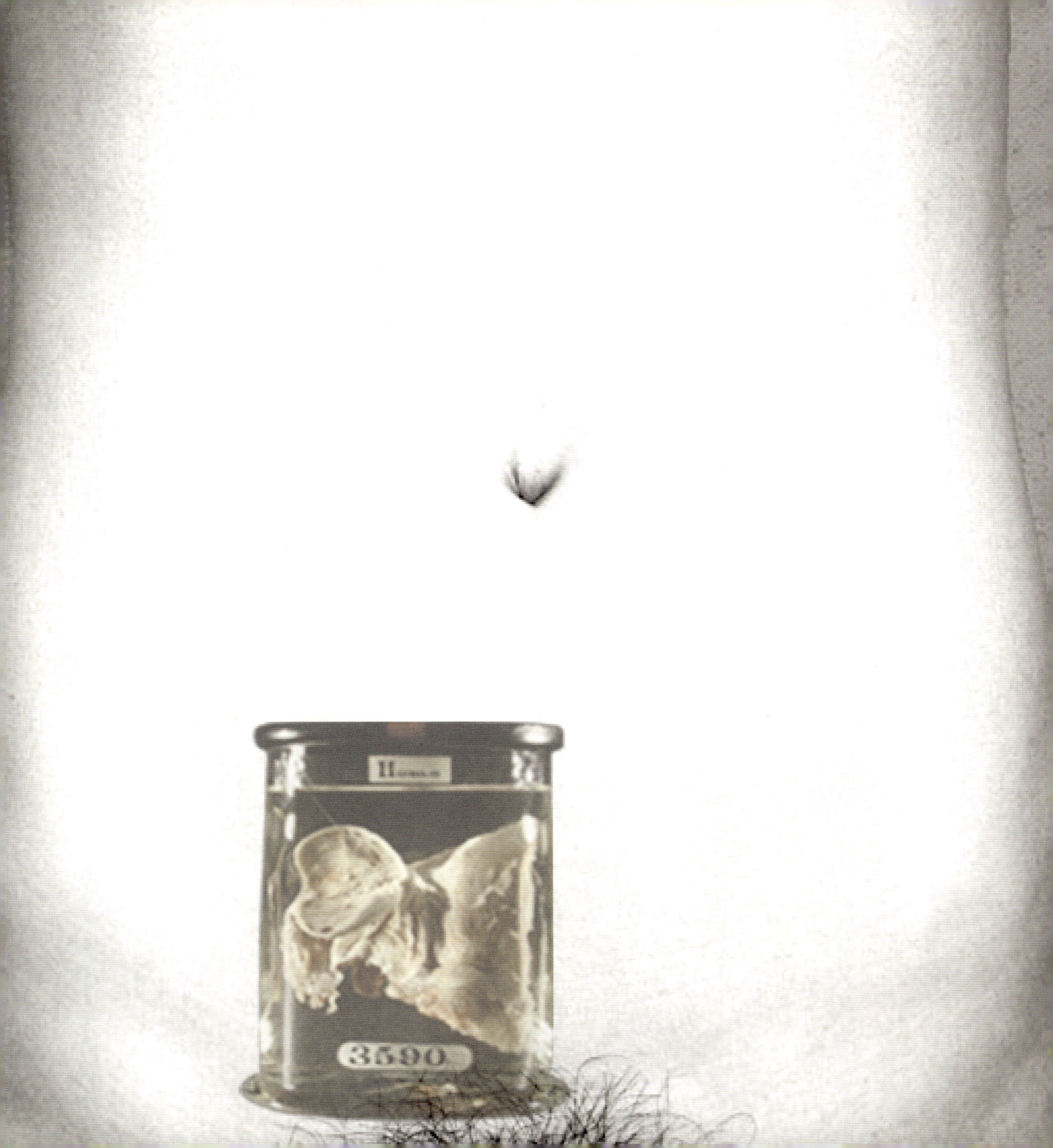
3590

RCSHC/3590

The left ovary, fallopian tube and half of the uterus from a woman in the first month of pregnancy. The ovary and fallopian tube have been opened and the cavity of the uterus has been exposed. The blood vessels have been injected. These specimens come from a woman aged 25. She was a domestic servant who committed suicide by taking poison. According to John Hunter, who carried out the post-mortem examination, she was pregnant, although her family suggested that her last period had been less than one month before. At the time it was suggested that the lateness of her period and the realisation that she was pregnant may have prompted her to take her own life.

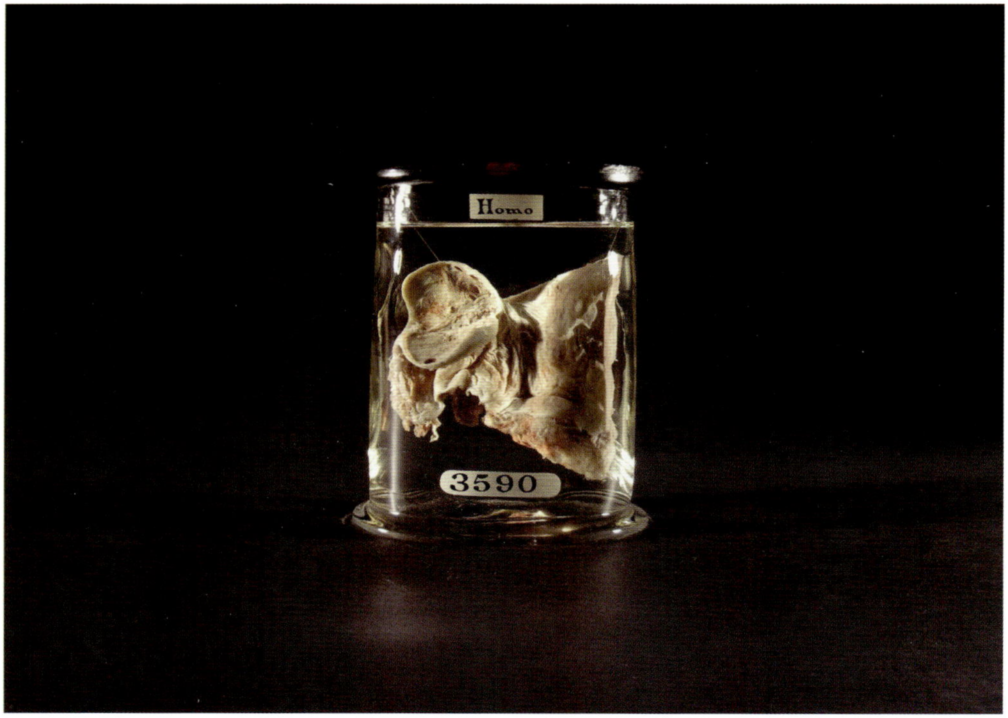

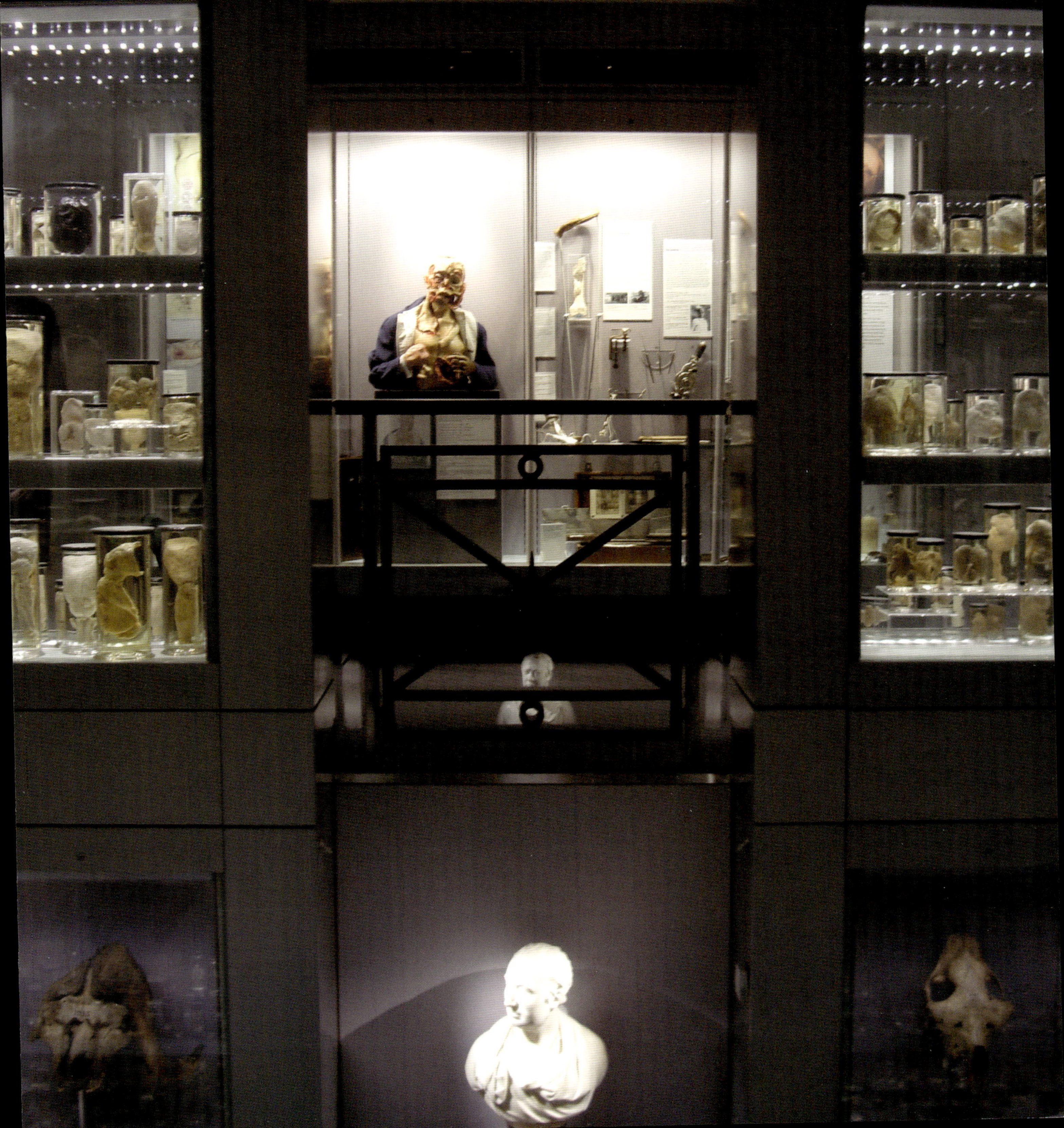

The Liver | RCSHC/P 1103

Margaret Johnson

“The pain, on the right side of the liver, would often be followed by convulsions and delirium. I drank gin and wine, already familiar helpmates to me, to ease my suffering. Ever larger quantities were needed, the respite being only temporary. Then the swelling, as if overnight some imp had stealthily filled me with water till I was fit to burst. Finally, the bleeding, until consciousness was lost and never regained. They blamed the drink for the damage (and there was me thinking it a help!). Perhaps my case will help some other poor soul, who in ignorance or desperation seeks solace in the drink. Meanwhile, here I am, properly pickled in my very own jar.”

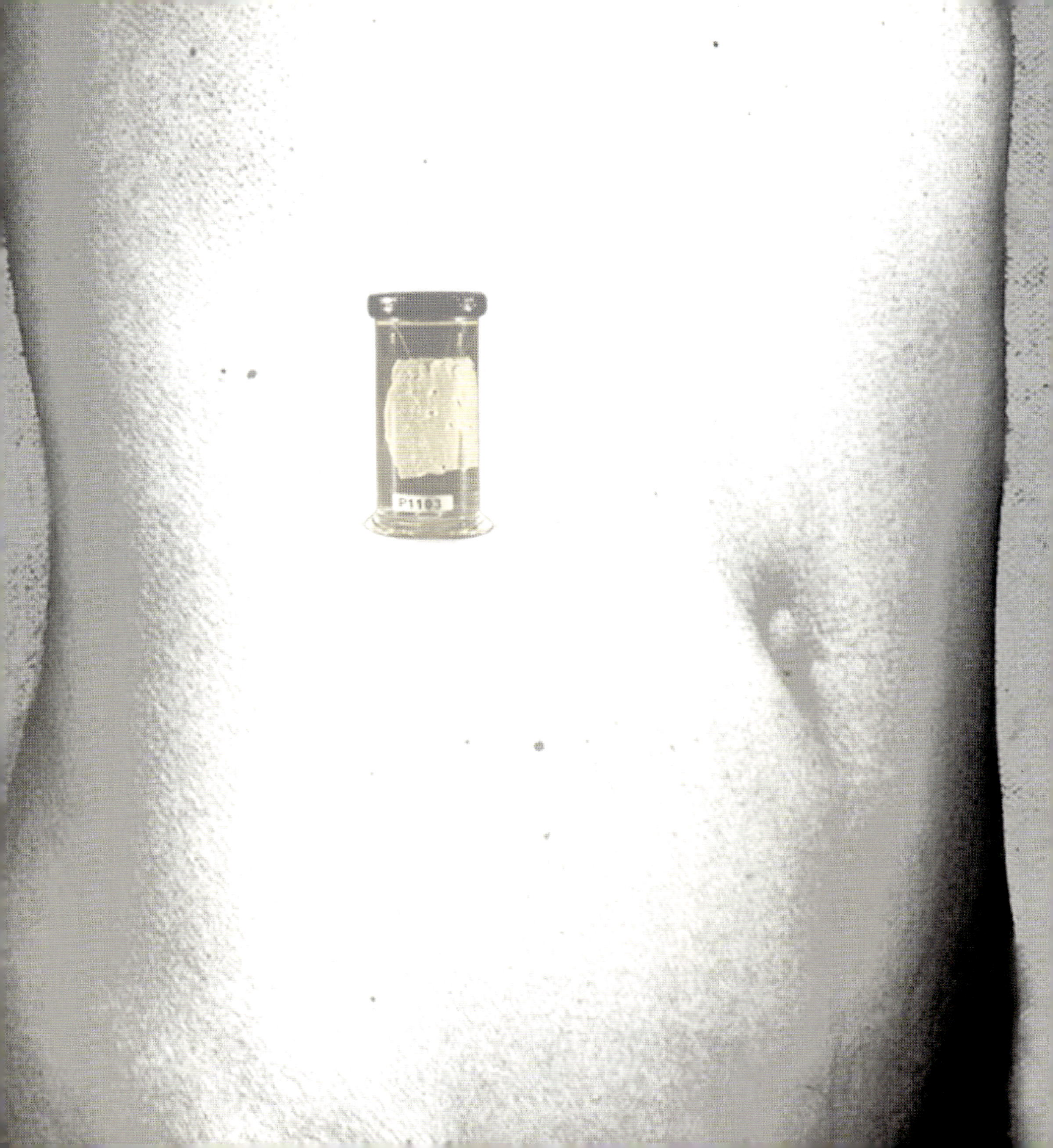
P1103

RCSHC/P 1103

A section of a liver showing changes to the substance of the organ as a result of cirrhosis. The tissue of the liver is pale, hardened and contracted. Round and oval nodules of fat project from the external surface of the liver. On the cut surface fibrous septa can be seen between these nodules. This preparation is believed to show alcoholic cirrhosis of the liver. The patient in this case was probably Margaret Johnston, a spinster, on whom John Hunter carried out a post-mortem in February 1760 at the request of the physician John Pringle.

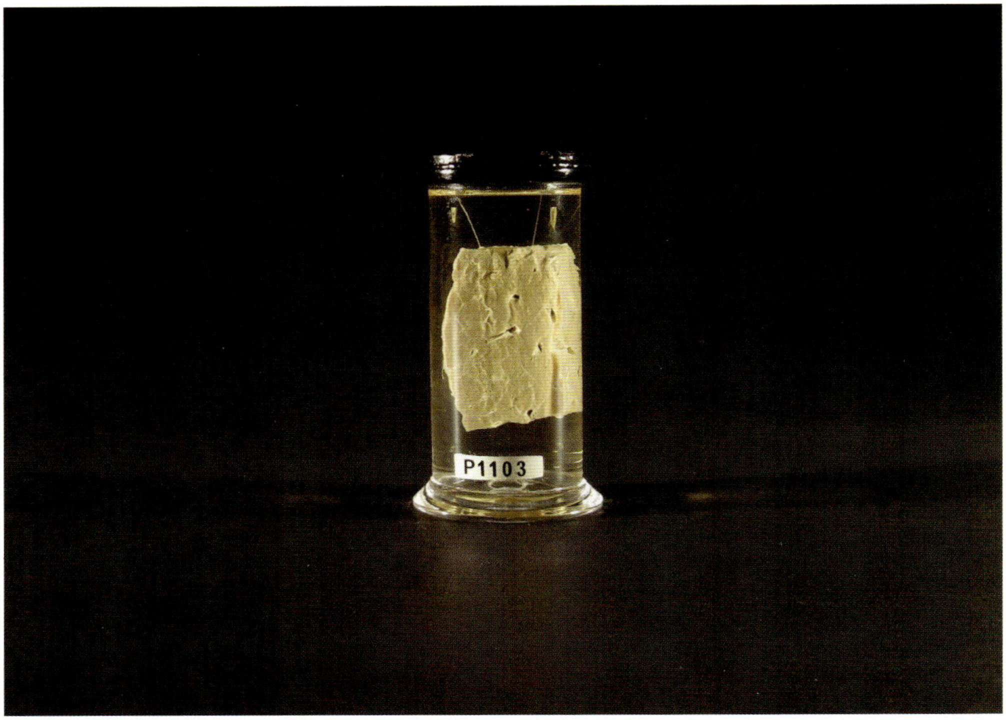

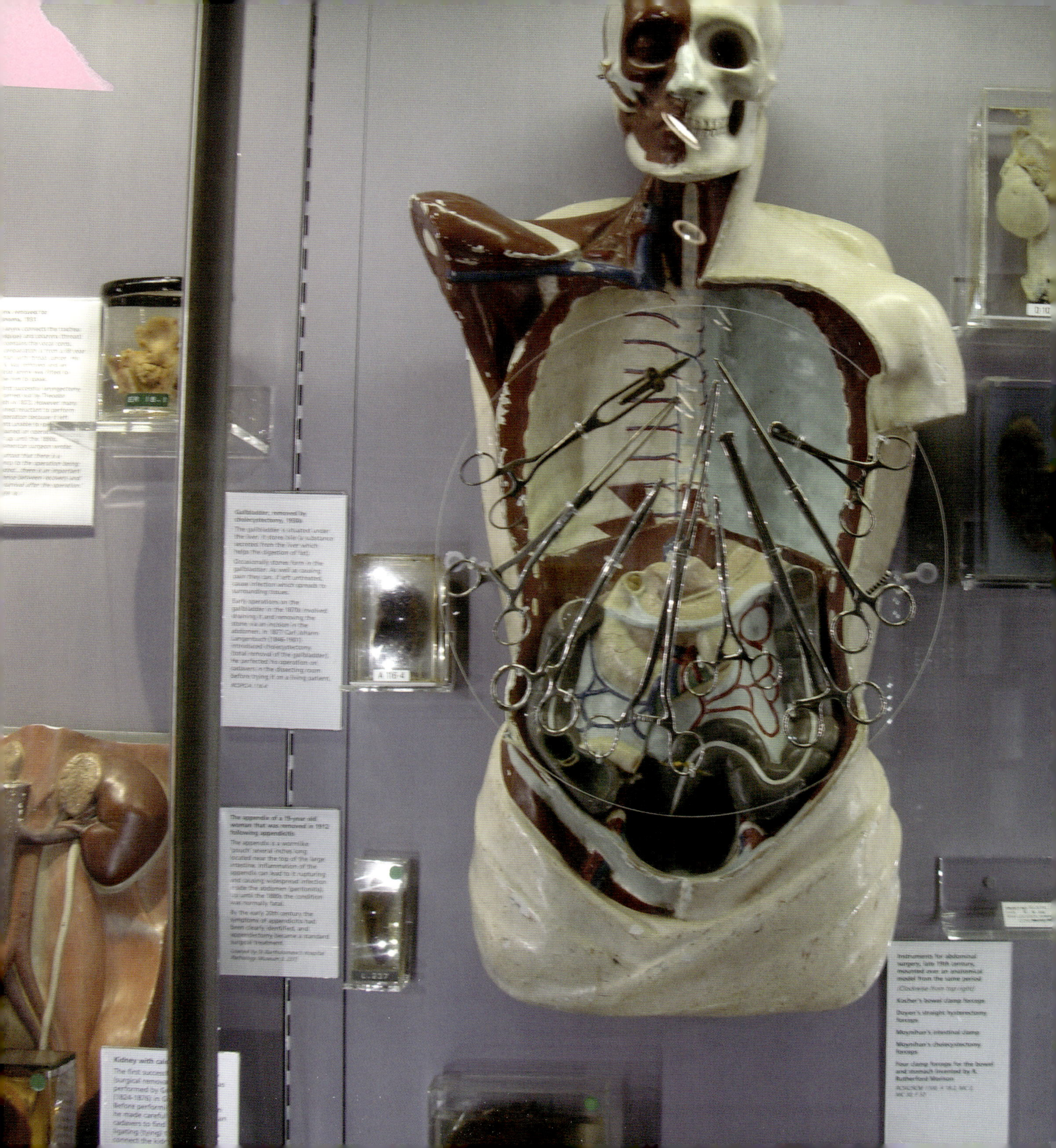
Instruments for abdominal surgery, late 19th century, mounted over an anatomical model from the same period
Kocher's bowel clamp forceps
Doyen's straight hysterectomy forceps
Moynihan's intestinal clamp
Moynihan's cholecystectomy forceps

The Lung | RCSHC/P 190
Mrs. Adam

"Such fine breasts, my husband was fond of saying, and I would titter like a girl. I should have known better than to delay, watching the lump swell and harden, but it seemed such a trifle at first. After examining me Mr. Hunter wanted to remove it, and with it my entire breast! But I procrastinated, and so he put the leeches to work, though little was the good they did me. Perhaps it was the fear of the operation, for fearful I was, anxious that the pain would be too much to bear. Perhaps it was not wanting to lose that part of me that defined me as a woman. Whatever the reason, when at last he operated it was too late. It seemed the cancer had spread to my lungs, strangling the very breath of me. Breath that became laboured and painful, until it did not come at all. What remains is what you see before you now, sealed in an airtight jar, the breath of life extinguished. And to think, had I acted with resolve, it might have been my fine breast that hung before you, while the breath of me, continued elsewhere."

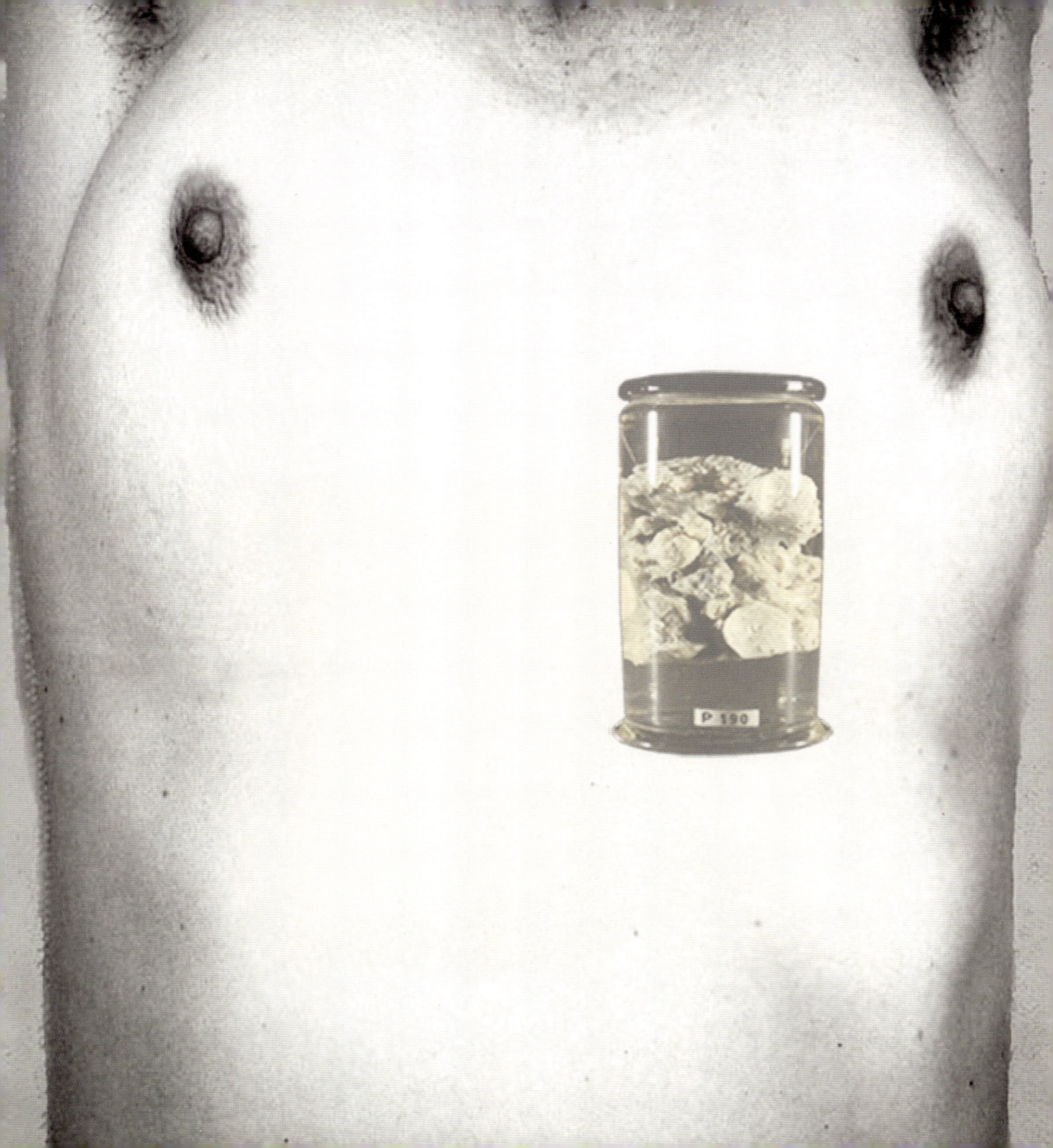
P 190

RCSHC/P 190

Portion of lung showing several round masses of firm white cancerous tissue embedded in apparently healthy pulmonary tissue. The neoplasms seen in the lung would have spread from a chondrosarcoma, whose primary site may have been the breast. The patient was a Mrs Adam, a woman aged about 40, who was treated by John Hunter for breast cancer. She initially refused his advice for removal of the breast. When she eventually agreed Hunter carried out the mastectomy, but by that stage the cancer had spread to the lung. She died three weeks after the operation.

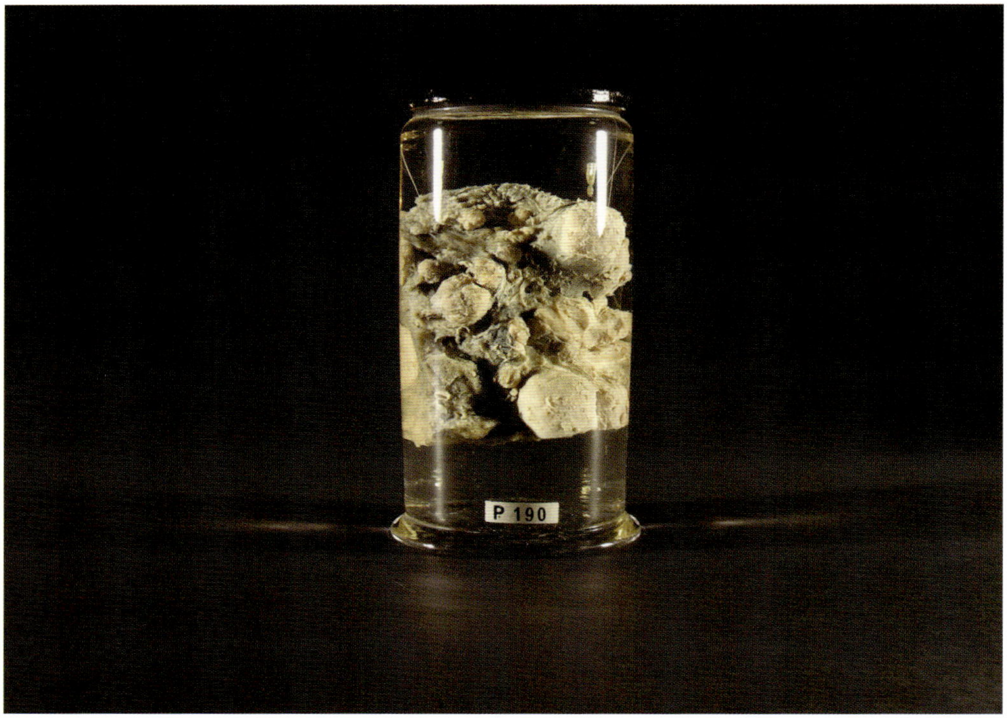

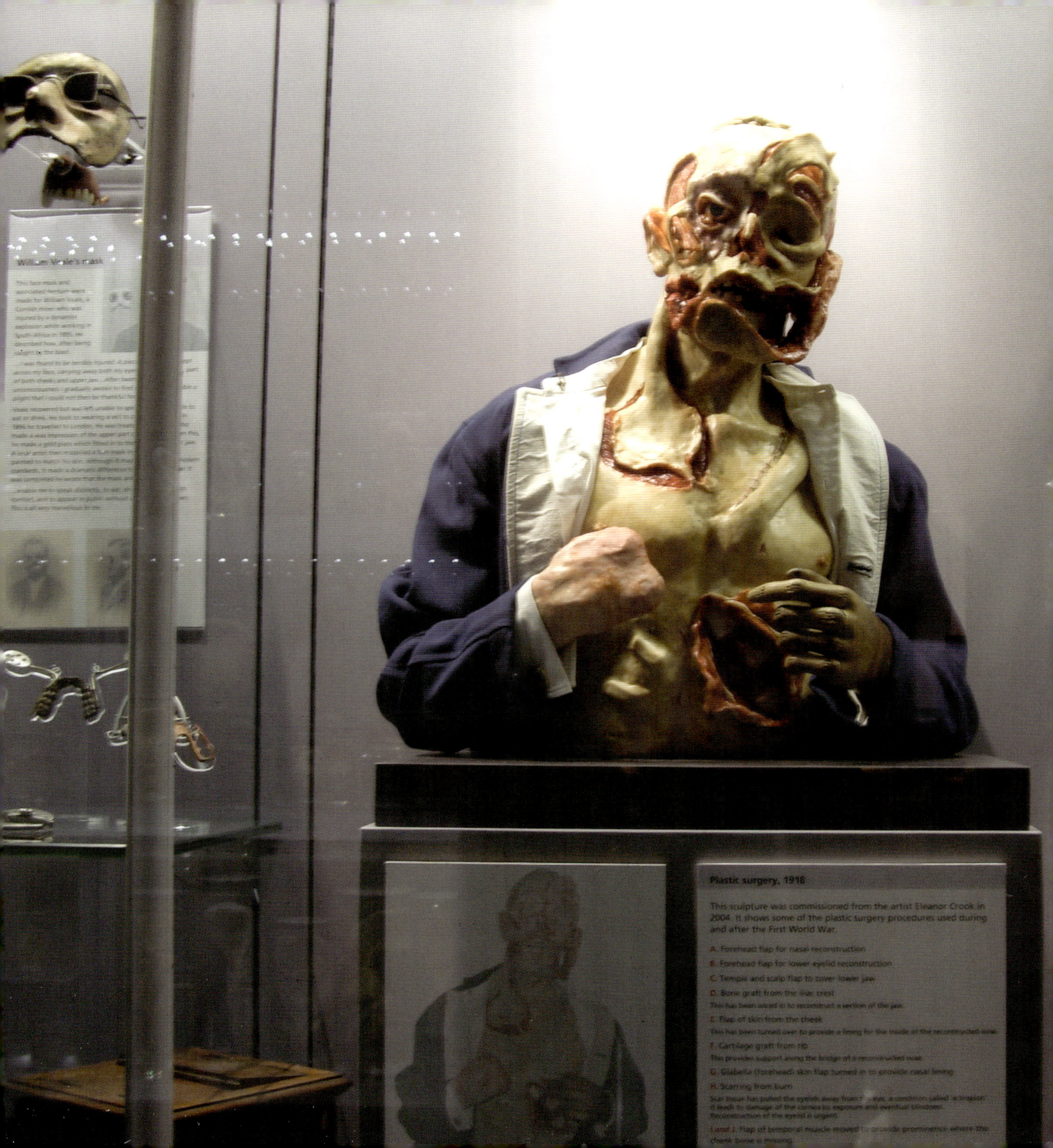
William Veale's mask
Plastic surgery, 1918
This sculpture was commissioned from the artist Eleanor Crook in 2004. It shows some of the plastic surgery procedures used during and after the First World War.
A. Forehead flap for nasal reconstruction
B. Forehead flap for lower eyelid reconstruction
C. Temple and scalp flap to cover lower jaw
D. Bone graft from the iliac crest
This has been wired in to reconstruct a section of the jaw.
E. Flap of skin from the cheek
This has been turned over to provide a lining for the inside of the reconstructed nose.
F. Cartilage graft from rib
This provides support along the bridge of a reconstructed nose.
G. Glabella (forehead) skin flap turned in to provide nasal lining
H. Scarring from burn

The Rectum | RCSHC/P 192

Thomas Thurlow - The Bishop of Durham

"Turtle soup, fillet of beef and ox tongue pie accompanied by a flagon of wine with port and cheese to follow. When in robust health these victuals had fed my body as the word of God fed my soul. But how I suffered their passage! The pain, the bloating and bleeding, at times copious; how they debilitated me. Thinking it a return of the piles I took Ward's Paste, which had proved so efficacious on previous occasions. But it was not to be. I knew from the graveness of Hunter's countenance that the news was bad: the disease commonly known as cancer. As I hang suspended here now, I think of those things that caused me such pleasure and pain; no longer food for the body, for save this part of me the body has long since gone, but merely food for thought."

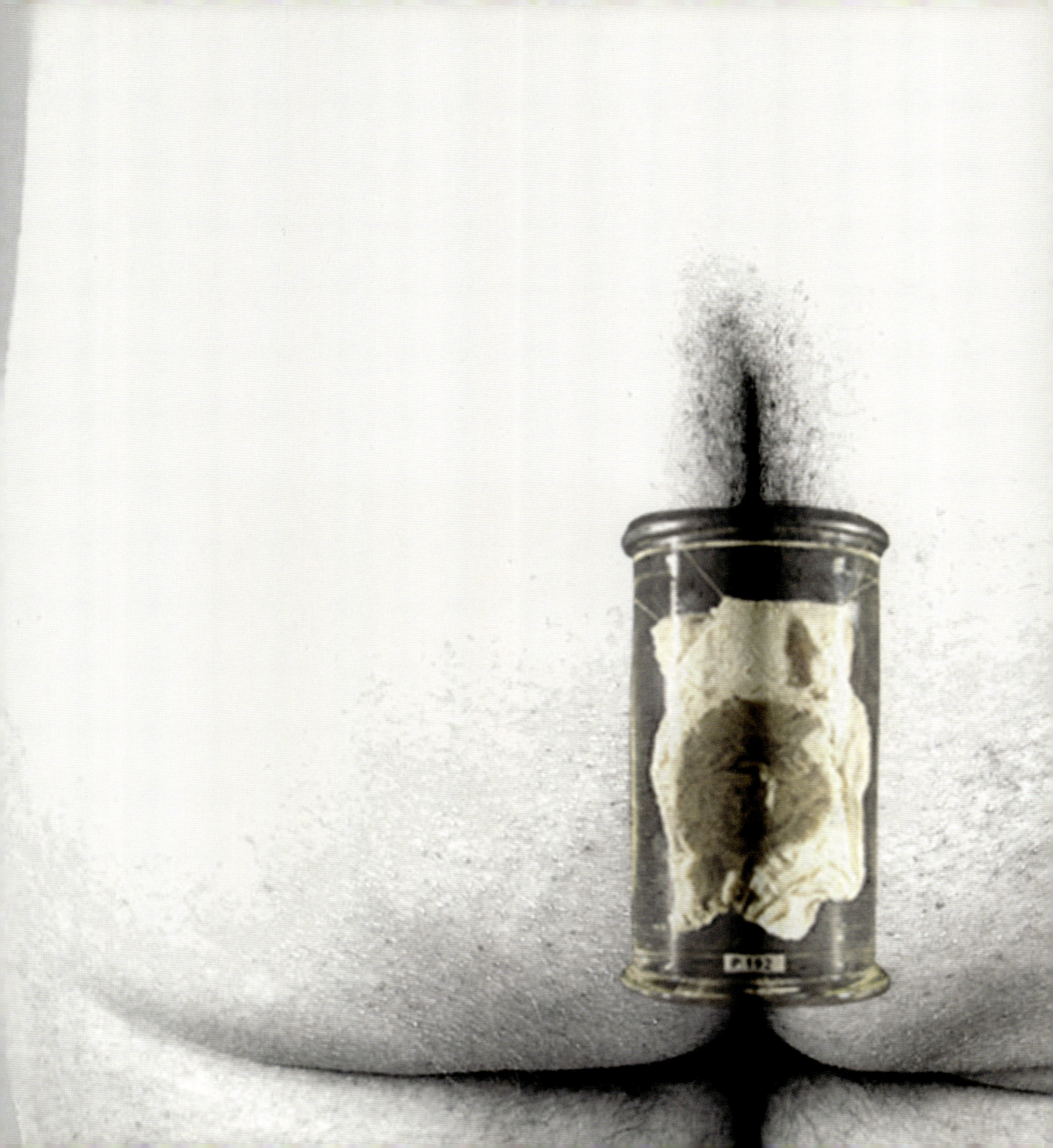

RCSHC/P 192

A rectum showing the effects of both haemorrhoids and bowel cancer. The patient in this case was Thomas Thurlow (1737-1791), the Bishop of Durham. Thurlow had suffered from some time from a bowel complaint which he initially thought was the result of piles. He consulted John Hunter after a number of other physicians and surgeons had failed to provide him with a satisfactory diagnosis. Hunter successfully identified the tumour through rectal examination but recognised that it was incurable. Thurlow died ten months later.

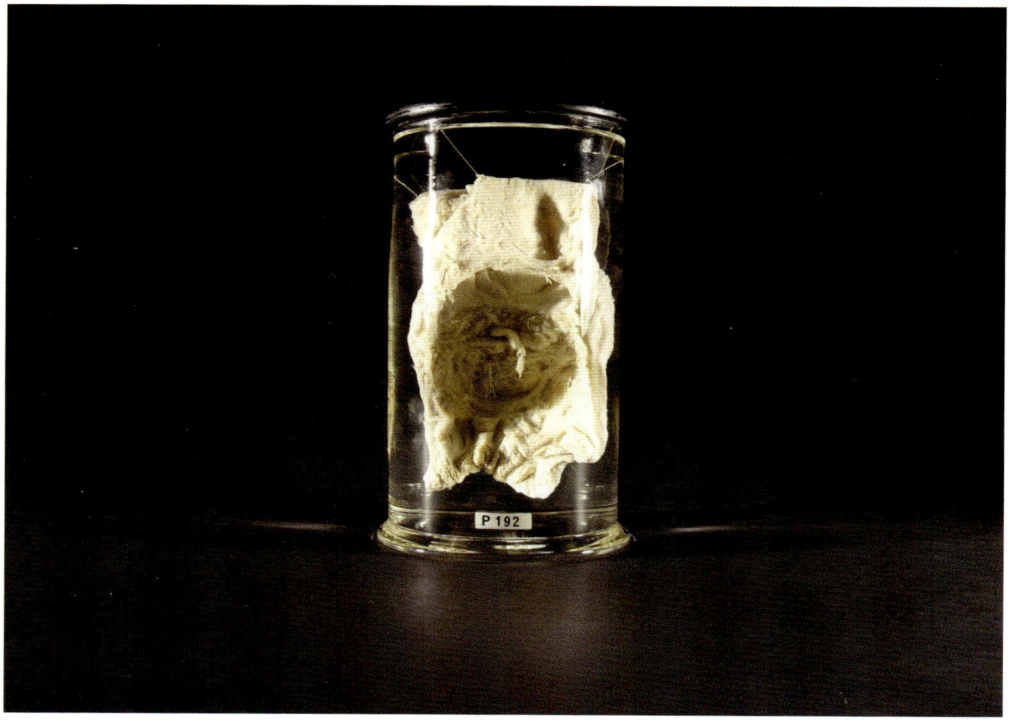

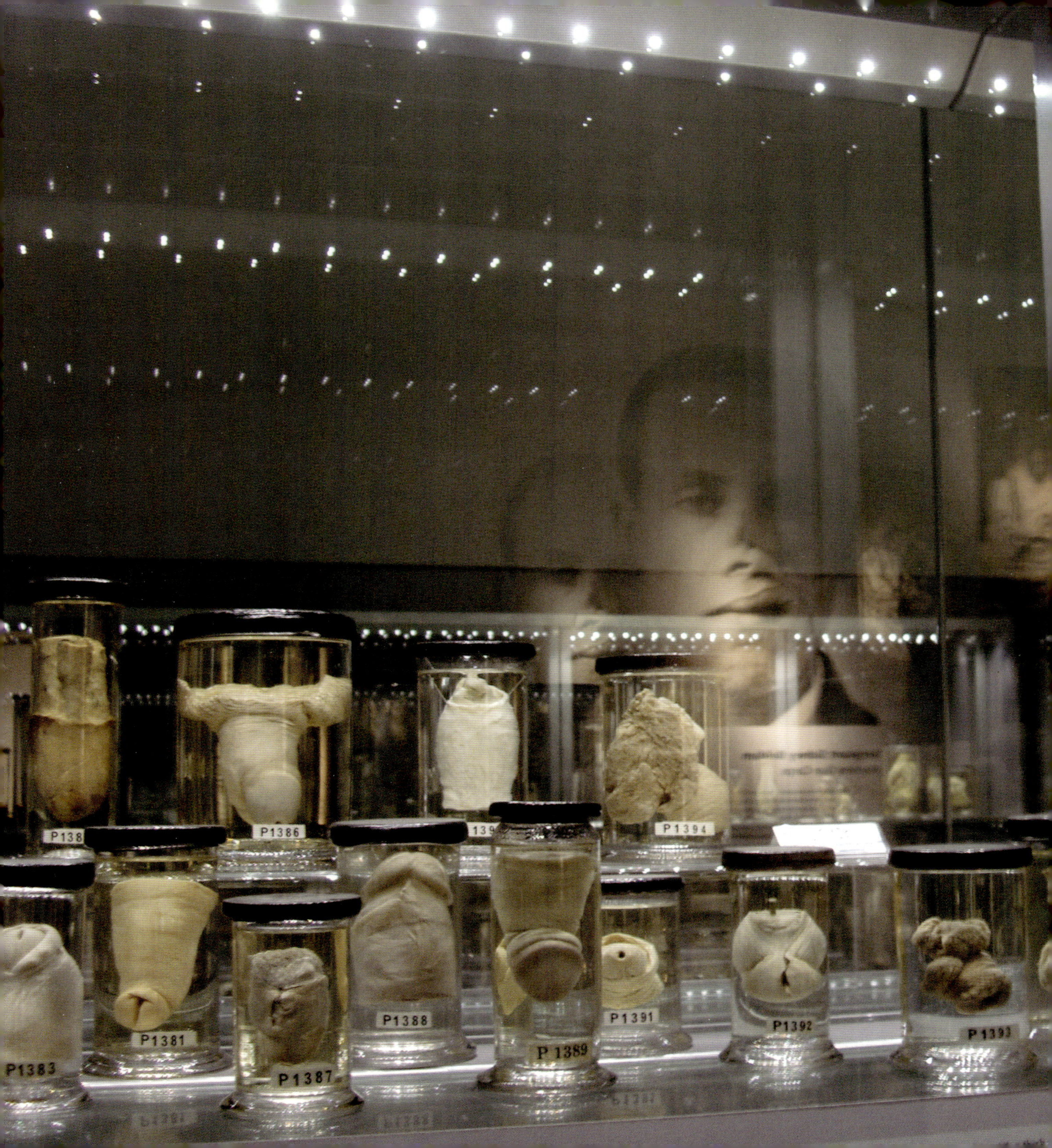
P1386
P1394
P1381
P1388
P 1389
P1391
P1392
P1393
P1383
P1387

The Heart | RCSHC/P 286
Richard Bulstrode

"They said I lacked courage and spirit, the boys who would taunt and tease me. I knew them to be wrong, but however much I strived to keep up, my weakened heart would let me down. Skipping and beating, palpitations so strong you could hear them, and the breath, when it came, painful and spare to the point of denial. My pride would not let it go, the taunts and derision. I took up the chase with a vengeance, letting my horse do the running and breathing for me, or so I thought. But the chase took its toll and in time I was abed, ridden with fever and fits of coughing. The bloodletting helped at first but all too soon the feeble beating of my heart was stilled. Holding my stagnant heart in his hands, this heart before you now, Hunter commented that the defects had likely been with me since infancy. Had it been otherwise it would have been a very fine heart. And so perhaps in death my pride, if not my health, has been somewhat restored."

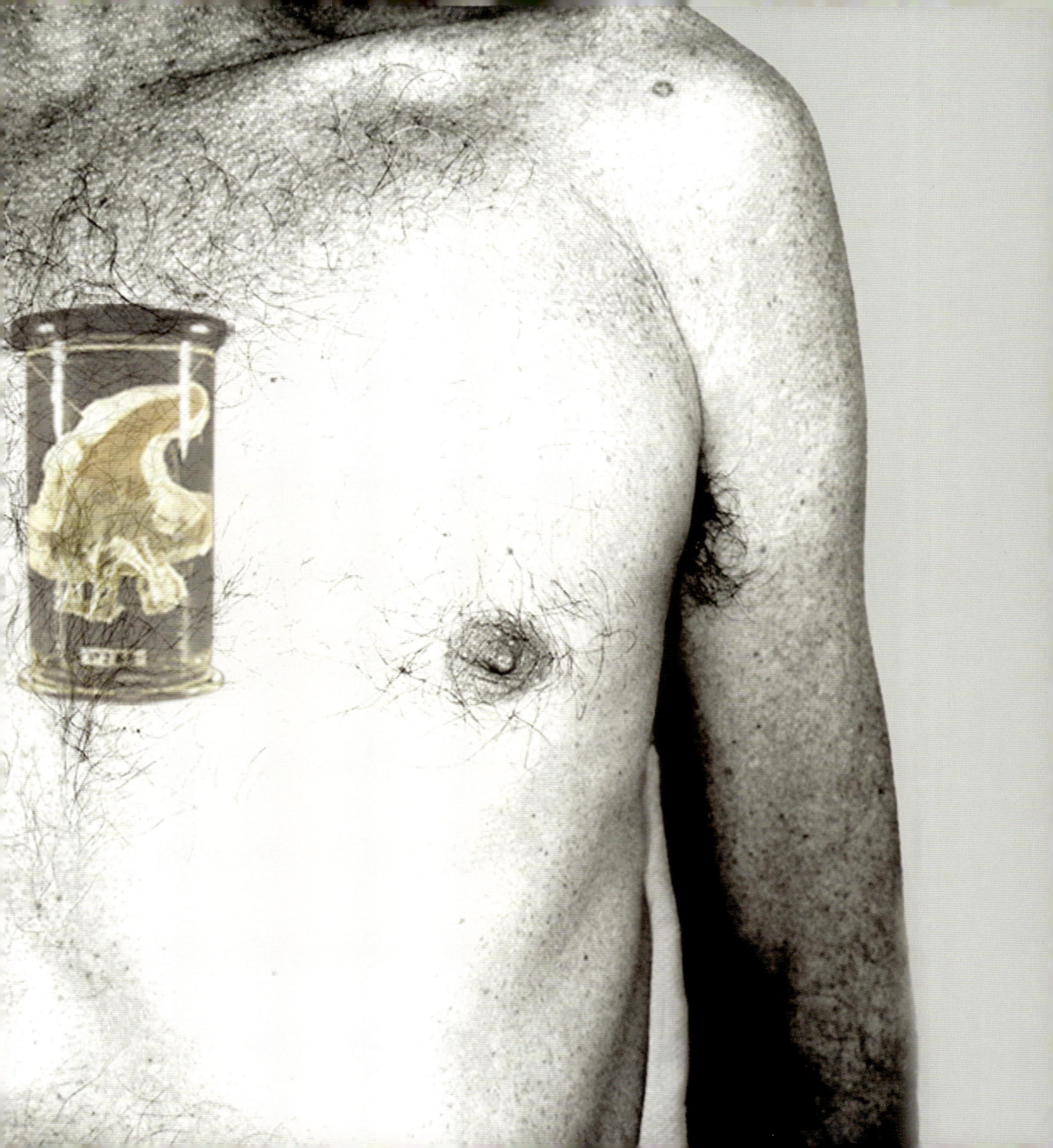

RCSHC/P 286

The mitral and aortic valves of the heart with adjacent parts showing the effects of rheumatic fever and endocarditis. The mitral valves are thickened with vegetations on the surfaces and rigid borders as a result of inflammation, while the aortic valves are shrivelled with backward curving and irregularly thickened margins. Both valves show a narrowing of their vessels due to rheumatic fever. The patient was a gentleman called Richard Bulstrode who had suffered from heart palpitations since infancy. In describing his case, Hunter mentioned that he 'solicited to open' [the body] after Bulstrode's death. This is one of several examples in which Hunter noted gaining permission from a patient's family to carry out a post-mortem, and to retain specimens from the body.

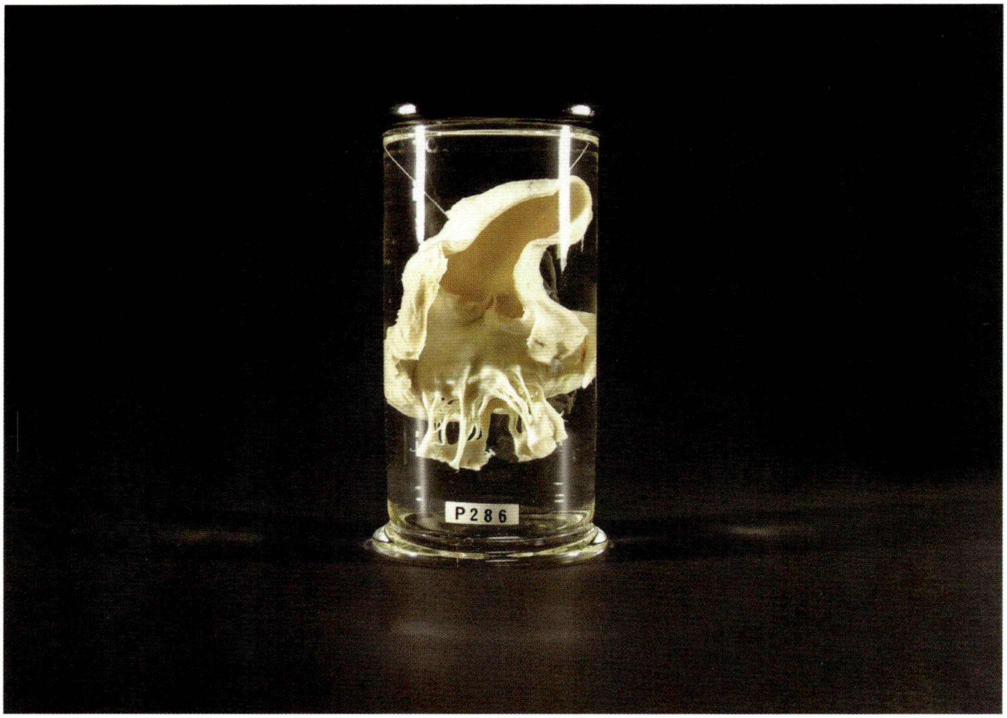

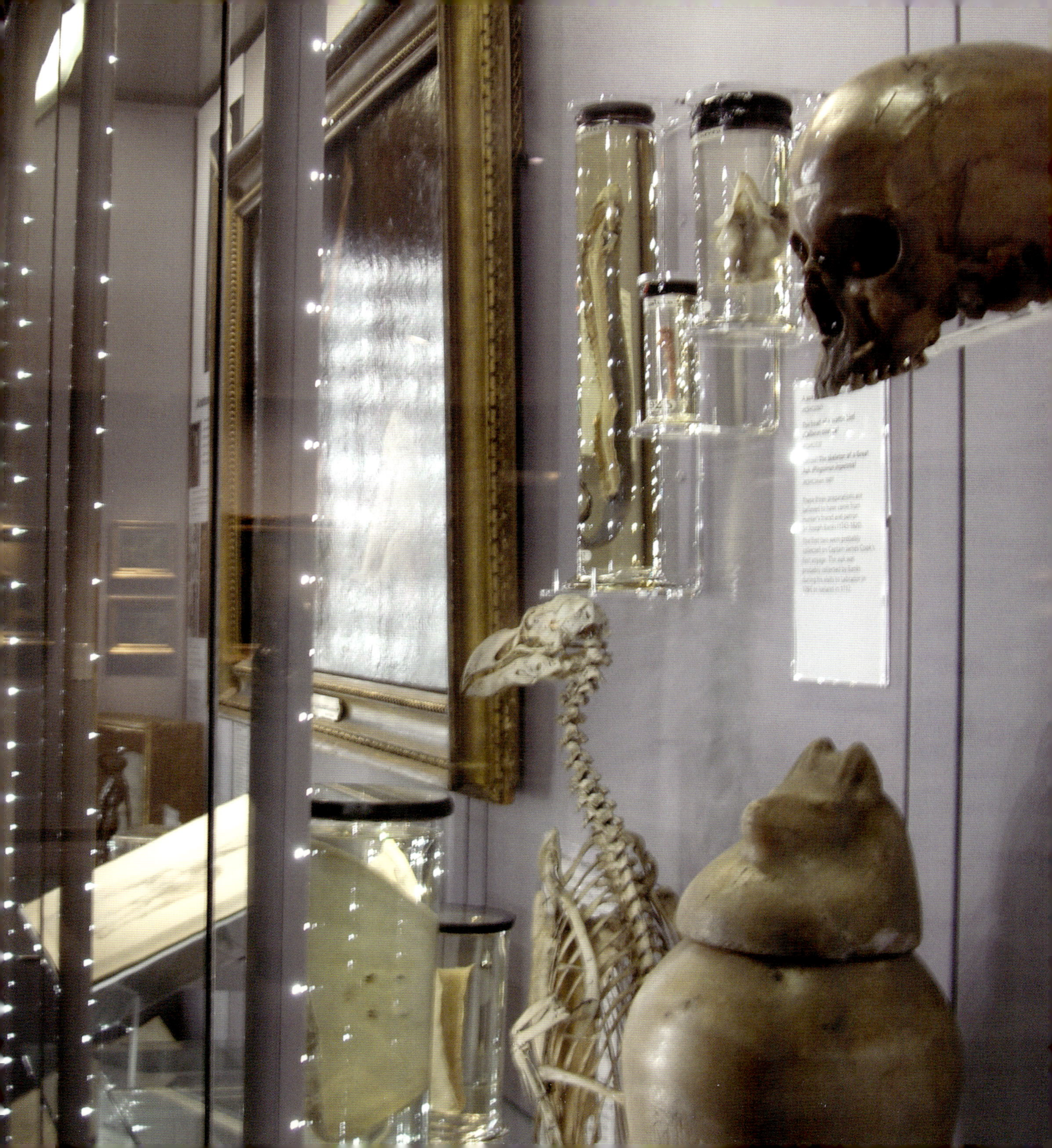

The Throat | RCSHC/P 364

Marianne Harland

"Not a sound. Not a whisper. Nothing escapes the tortured confines of my diseased throat. Where once there was song there is now only rasping. Where once there was speech, silence. Where once there was beauty, pain. My young son will never experience the famed delights of his mother's pure, clear, choral range, nor will he hear me speak his name. I cannot even utter the name of my killer, no more than the doctors could halt the all too rapid progress of this dreadful disease. And now I am enclosed in a world of perpetual silence, my throat opened and displayed for all the world to see. All that is left of me. Not a song. Not a whisper."

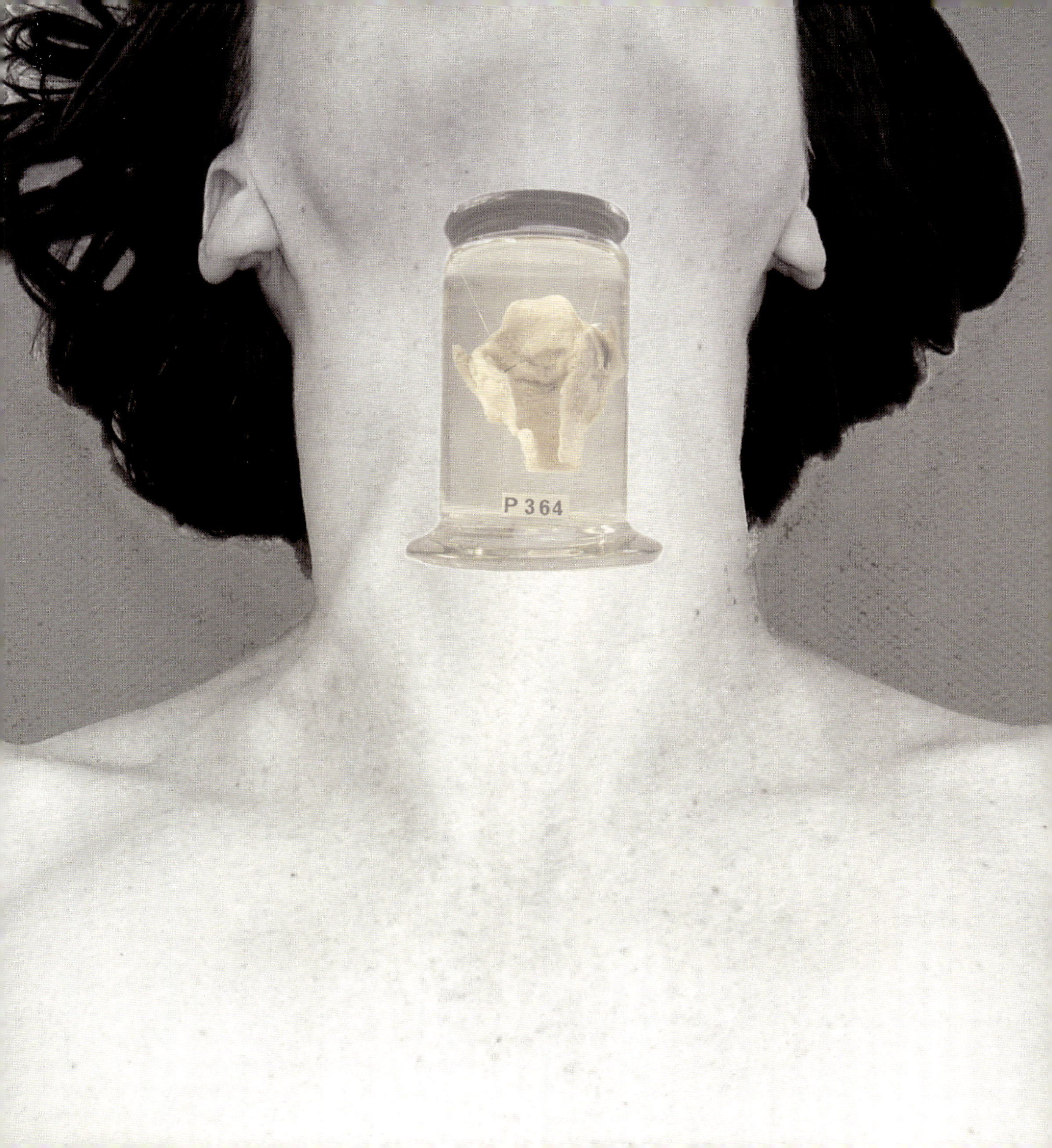
P 364

RCSHC/P 364

A larynx and trachea showing changes consistent with tuberculosis. The mucous membrane of the larynx has ulcerated, being diffuse and irregular around the vocal chords. The ulcerations are in places deep enough to have exposed ossified arytenoid cartilage. The patient in this case was Marianne Dorothy Dalrymple, née Harland (1756-1785). Hunter remarked that Harland was known for her musical talents and singing voice. This is reflected in a portrait of her by Richard Cosway (1742-1821) which shows her playing a harp and surrounded by other musical instruments. Her death from a disease of the throat therefore carried with it even greater poignancy, a quality that was probably not lost on the visitors to John Hunter's museum who included many of the regular guests for Anne Hunter's musical and literary salons.

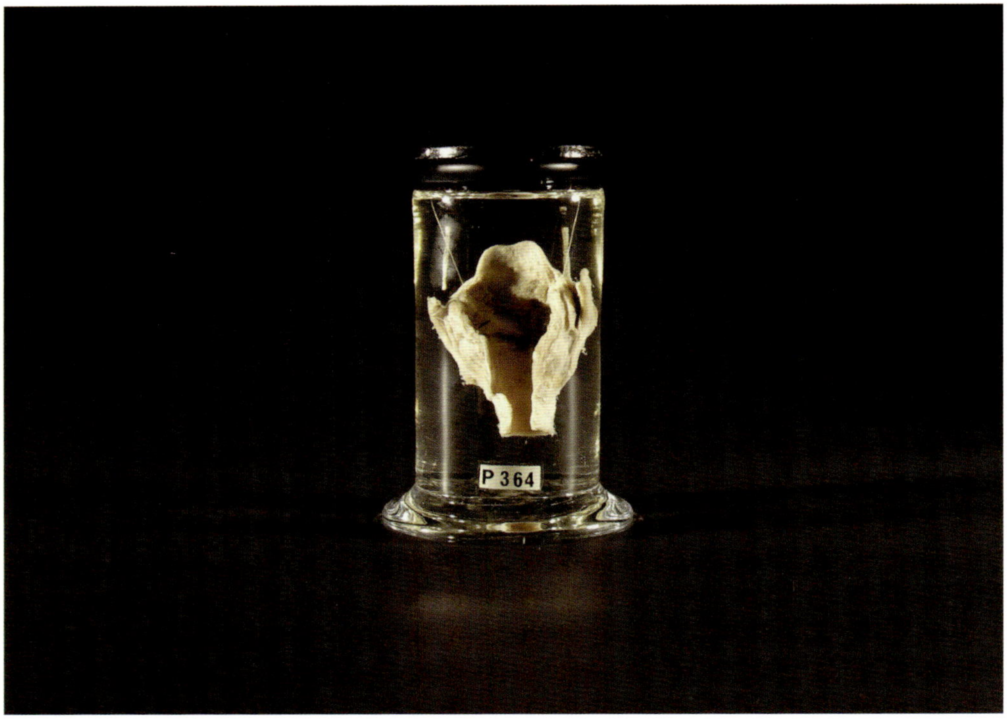

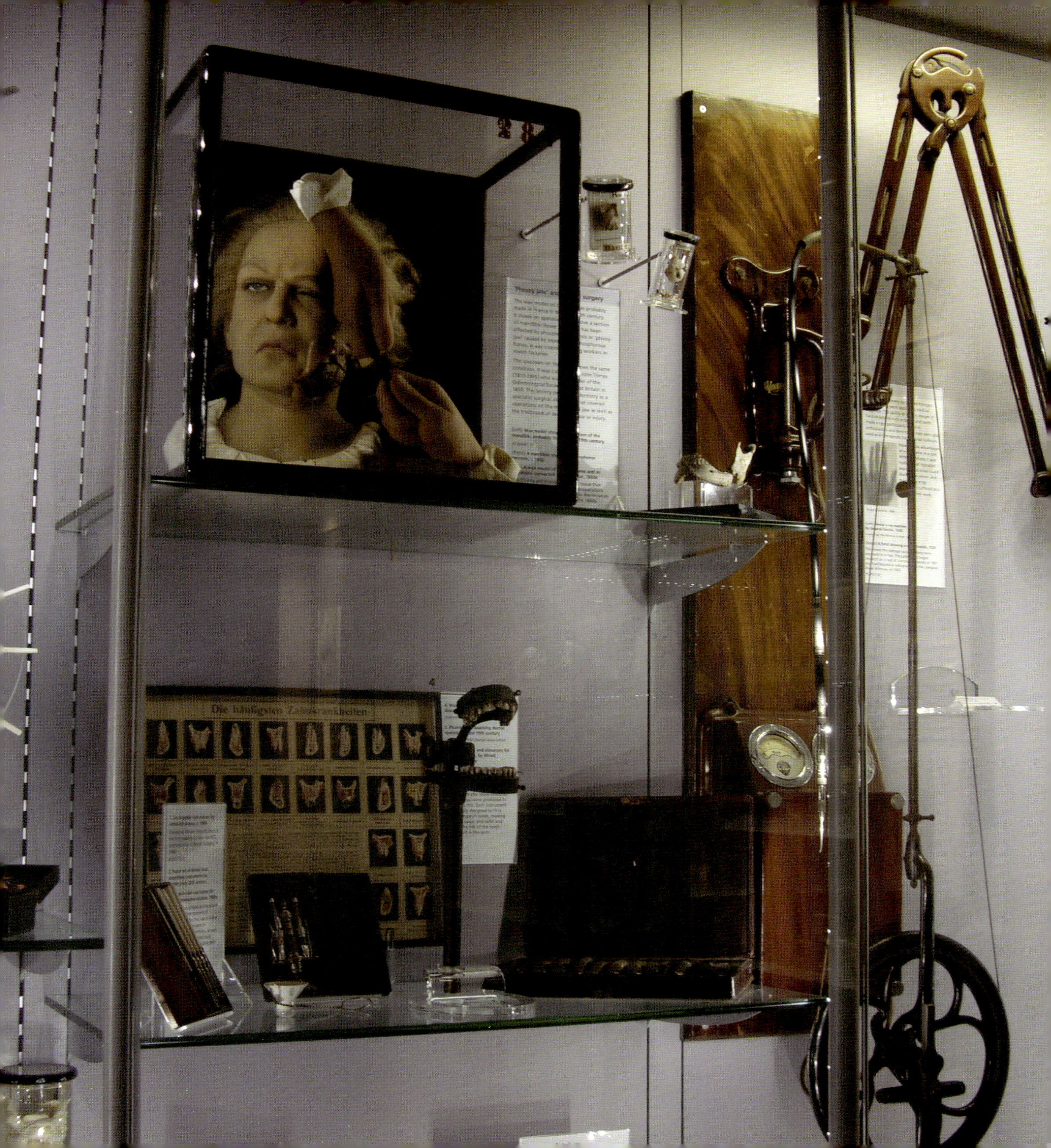
Die häufigsten Zahnkrankheiten

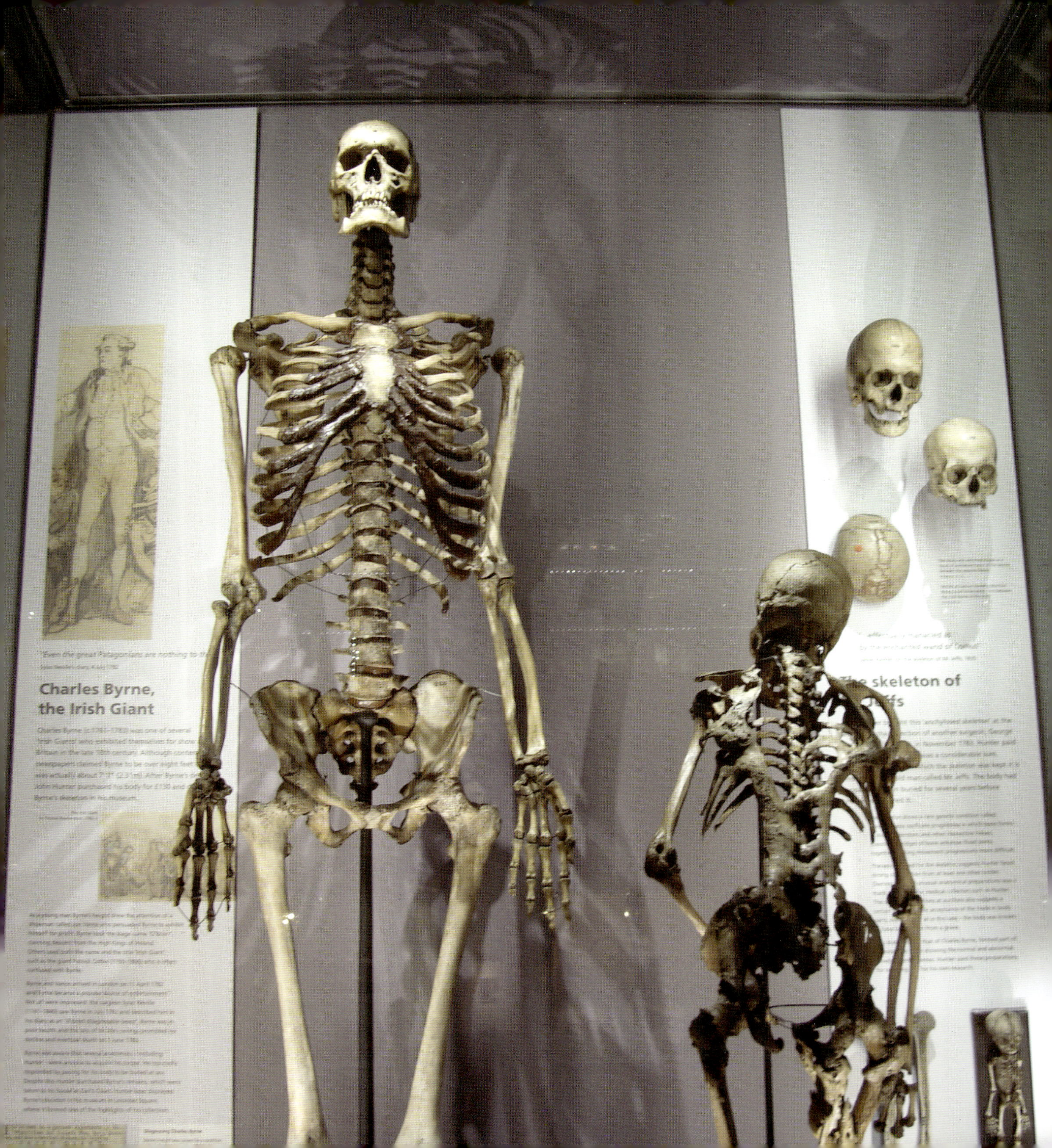
Charles Byrne,
the Irish Giant
The skeleton of

Acknowledgements

Narrative Remains is the result of a process of creative collaboration and negotiation and as such there are many individuals and institutions that have contributed to the projects realisation. I would like to thank The Wellcome Trust Arts Awards for their support and also the Royal College of Surgeons of England Hunterian Museum in London's Lincoln's Inn Fields. In particular I owe a debt of thanks to the museum's director Simon Chaplin for his enthusiasm, knowledge, and willingness to trust in the artistic and collaborative process, and for his insightful essay. The support of the Dynevor Centre for Art, Design and Media is also greatly appreciated and I would like to thank Andrea Liggins, Howard Riley, Manolo Lozano, James Morgan, Tim Stokes, Andrew Hamley, Sarah Tierney, Bella Kerr, Angela Maddock, Sue Griffith, Hamish Gane, and Phil Thomas for their support and contributions. Extract from 'Love Bite' by Kathryn Ashill courtesy of the artist. Extract from 'Pregnant Pauses' by James Morgan courtesy of the artist.

First published in the UK in 2009

ISBN: 978-0-9561003-1-3

http://www.karenigham.org.uk/
narrative remains

Design: Phil Thomas

wellcome trust

Hunterian Museum
Royal College of Surgeons

CLASI